Volume 3

The National Diet and Nutrition Survey:
Headline results from Years 1, 2 and 3 (combined)
of the rolling programme, 2008/9 - 2010/11

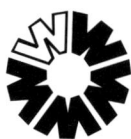

NatCen
National Centre for Social Research

UCL

MRC | Human Nutrition Research

NATIONAL DIET AND NUTRITION SURVEY

Food and Drink Diary

DIARY START DATE: _____

CKL ☐

RESPONDENT No ☐

SERIAL NUMBER ☐☐☐☐☐☐☐

FIRST NAME ☐☐☐☐☐☐

Date of birth: ☐☐☐☐☐☐

Sex: Male / Female

INTERVIEWER NUMBER: ☐☐☐☐

INTERVIEWER NAME: ☐

NDNS (I) Diary_Adult_A4, April 09 REC Ref. 07/H0604/113

For use from 01/04/10

NATIONAL DIET AND NUTRITION SURVEY

Food and Drink Diary

If you have any queries about how to complete the diary please contact a member of the NDNS Team at NatCen on freephone **0800 652 4572** between 8.30am-5.30pm.

PLEASE READ THROUGH THESE PAGES BEFORE STARTING YOUR DIARY

We would like you to keep this diary of _everything you eat and drink_ over 4 days. Please include all food consumed at home and outside the home e.g. work, college or restaurants. It is very important that you do not change what you normally eat and drink just because you are keeping this record. Please keep to your usual food habits.

Day and Date
Please write down the day and date at the top of the page each time you start a new day of recording.

Time Slots
Please note the time of each eating occasion into the space provided. For easy use each day is divided into sections, from the first thing in the morning to late evening and through the night.

Where and with whom?
For each eating occasion, please tell us what **room or part of the house** you were in when you ate, e.g. kitchen, living room, If you ate at your work canteen, a restaurant, fast food chain or your car, write that location down. We would also like to know **who you share your meals with**, e.g. whether you ate alone or with others. If you ate with others please describe their relationship to you e.g. partner, children, colleagues, or friends. We would also like to know **when you ate at a table** and **when you were watching television whilst eating.** For those occasions where you were **not** at a table or watching TV please write 'Not at table' or 'No TV' rather than leaving it blank.

What do you eat?
Please describe the food you eat in as much detail as possible. Be as specific as you can. Pages 16 - 21 will help with the sort of detail we need, like **cooking methods** (fried, grilled, baked etc) and any **additions** (fats, sugar/sweeteners, sauces, pepper etc).

☐ **Homemade dishes**

If you have eaten any **homemade dishes** e.g. chicken casserole, please record the name of the recipe, ingredients with amounts (including water or other fluids) for the whole recipe, the number of people the recipe serves, and the cooking method. Write this down in the recipe section at the end of the record day. Record how much of the whole recipe you have eaten in the portion size column (see examples on pages 4 - 15).

☐ **Take-aways and eating out**

If you have eaten **take-aways** or **made up dishes not prepared at home** such as at a restaurant or a friend's house, please record as much detail about the ingredients as you can e.g. vegetable curry containing chickpeas, aubergine, onion and tomato.

Brand name
Please note the **brand name** (if known). Most packed foods will list a brand name, e.g. Bird's eye, Hovis, or Supermarket own brands.

☐ _Labels/Wrappers_

Labels are an important source of information for us. It helps us a great deal if you enclose, in the plastic bag provided, labels from all **ready meals**, labels from **foods of lesser known brands** and also from any **supplements** you take.

Portion sizes

Examples for how to describe the **quantity** or **portion size** you had of a particular food or drink are shown on pages 16 - 21.

For foods, quantity can be described using:

- **household measures,** e.g. one teaspoon (tsp) of sugar, two thick slices of bread, 4 tablespoons (tbsp) of peas, ½ cup of gravy. Be careful when describing amounts in spoons that you are referring to the correct spoon size. Compare the spoons you use with the life size pictures at the back of this diary.
- **weights from labels,** e.g. 4oz steak, 420g tin of baked beans, 125g pot of yoghurt
- **number of items,** e.g. 4 fish fingers, 2 pieces of chicken nuggets, 1 regular size jam filled doughnut
- **picture examples** for specific foods on pages 22-24.

For drinks, quantity can be described using:

- the **size of glass, cup etc** (e.g. large glass) or the **volume** (e.g. 300ml). Examples of typical drinks containers are on pages 26-27.
- **volumes from labels** (e.g. 330ml can of fizzy drink).

We would like to know the **amount that was actually eaten** which means taking **leftovers** into account. You can do this in two ways:

1. Record what was served and make notes of what was not eaten e.g. 3 tbsp of peas, only 2 tbsp eaten; 1 large sausage roll, ate only ½
2. Only record the amount actually eaten i.e. 2 tbsp of peas, ½ a large sausage roll

Was it a typical day?

After each day of recording you will be prompted to tell us whether this was a typical day or whether there were any reasons why you ate and drank more or less than usual.

Supplements

At the end of each recording day there is a section for providing information about any supplements you took. Brand name, full name of supplement, strength and the amount taken should be recorded.

When to fill in the diary

Please record your eating as you go, not from memory at the end of the day. Use written notes on a pad if you forget to take your diary with you. Each diary day covers a 24hr period, so please include any food or drinks that you may have had during the night. Remember to include foods and drinks between meals (snacks) including water.

Overleaf you can see 2 example days that have been filled in by different people. These examples show you how we would like you to record your food and drink, for example a ready meal and a homemade dish. Your instruction booklet contains further examples such as how to describe food eaten in a restaurant.

It only takes a few minutes for each eating occasion!

For your convenience a separate booklet with instructions and examples is provided.

Thank you for your time – we really appreciate it!

Day: Thurs		Date: 31st March		
Time	**Where?** **With Whom?** **TV on?** **At table?**	**Food/Drink description & preparation**	**Brand Name**	**Portion size or** **quantity <u>eaten</u>**
		How to describe what you had and how much you had can be found on pages 16 - 21		
		6am to 9am		
6.30 am	Kitchen Alone No TV Not at table	Filter coffee, decaffeinated milk (fresh, semi-skimmed) Sugar white	Douwe Egberts Silverspoon	Mug A little 1 level tsp
7.30 am	Kitchen Partner TV on At table	Filter coffee with milk and sugar Cornflakes Milk (fresh, semi-skimmed) Toast, granary medium sliced Light spread Marmalade	As above Tesco's own Hovis Flora Hartleys	As above 1b drowned 1 slice med spread 1 heaped tsp
		9am to 12 noon		
10.15 am	Office desk Alone No TV Not at table	Instant coffee, not decaffeinated Milk (fresh, whole) Sugar brown	Kenco	Mug A little 1 level tsp
11 am	Office desk Alone No TV Not at table	Digestive biscuit – chocolate coated on one side	McVities	2

Time	Where? With Whom? TV on? At table?	Food/Drink description & preparation	Brand Name	Portion size or quantity eaten
		12 noon to 2pm		
12.30 pm	Tea room at work Colleagues No TV At table	Ham salad sandwich from home Bread, wholemeal, thick sliced Light spread Low fat Mayonnaise Smoked ham thinly sliced Lettuce, iceberg Cucumber with skin Unsweetened orange juice from canteen Apple with skin from home, Braeburn	Tesco's own Flora Hellmans Tesco's own Tropicana	2 slices thin spread on 1 slice 2 teaspoons 2 slices 1 leaf 4 thin slices 250ml carton medium size, core left
		2pm to 5pm		
3 pm	Meeting room at work With supervisor No TV Not at table	Tea, decaffeinated Milk (fresh, whole) Jaffa cake – mini variety	Twinings Tesco's own McVities	Mug Some 6

Time	Where? With Whom? TV on? At table?	Food/Drink description & preparation	Brand Name	Portion size or quantity eaten
		5pm to 8pm		
6.30 pm	Pub Partner TV on At table	Gin Tonic water diet Lager 3.8% alcohol Salted peanuts	Gordon's Schweppes Draught, Carlberg KP	Single measure 1/2 small glass 1 pint 1 handful
8 pm	Dining room Family No TV At table	Spaghetti, wholemeal Bolognese sauce (see recipe) Courgettes (fried in butter) Tinned peaches in juice (juice drained) Single cream UHT	Tesco's own Prince's	3b 6 tablespoons 4 tablespoons 3 halves 1 tablespoon
		Orange squash No Added Sugar	Sainsbury's own	200ml glass, 1 part squash, 3 parts tap water
		8pm to 10pm		
9 pm	Sitting room Alone TV on Not at table	Grapes, green, seedless Chocolates, chocolate creams Potato crisps, Prawn Cocktail	Bendicks Walkers	15 2 25g bag (from multipack)
		10pm to 6am		
10.30 pm	Bed room Partner No TV Not at table	Camomile tea (no milk or sugar)	Twinings	1 mug

Was the amount of **food** that you had today about what you usually have, less than usual, or more than usual?

Yes, usual [✓]

No, **less** than usual [ ]

No, **more** than usual [ ]

Please tell us why you had less than usual

Please tell us why you had more than usual

Was the amount you had to **drink** today, including water, tea, coffee and soft drinks [and alcohol], about what you usually have, less than usual, or more than usual?

Yes, usual [ ]

No, **less** than usual [ ]

No, **more** than usual [✓]

Please tell us why you had less than usual

Please tell us why you had more than usual

Went to pub after work

Did you **finish all the food and drink** that you recorded in the diary today?

Yes ☑   No ☐

If no, please **go back to the diary and make a note of any leftovers**

Did you take any **vitamins, minerals or other food supplements** today?

Yes ☑   No ☐

If yes, **please describe the supplements you took below**

Brand	Name (in full) including strength	Number of pills, capsules, teaspoons
Healthspan	Omega3 fish oil with vitamin A, C, D & E	2 capsules
Boots	Calcium (1000mg) with vitamin D	1 tablet
Holland & Barrett	Vitamin C 60mg	1 tablet

Please record over the page details of any recipes or (if not already described) ingredients of made up dishes or take-away dishes.

Write in recipes or ingredients of made up dishes or take-away dishes

NAME OF DISH: *Bolognese sauce*

SERVES: 4

Ingredients	Amount	Ingredients	Amount
Co-op low fat beef mince	500g	Lea & Perrins worcester sauce	dash
garlic	3 cloves		
onion	1 medium		
sweet red pepper	1 medium		
Napoli chopped tomatoes	400g tin		
Tesco tomato puree	1 tablespoon		
Tesco olive oil	1 tablespoon		
mixed herbs	1 dessertspoon		

Brief description of cooking method

Fry onion & garlic in oil, add mince and fry till brown.

Add pepper, tomatoes, puree, Worcester sauce & herbs. Simmer for 30 mins

Day:	Friday	Date: 28.09.2007		
Time	Where? With Whom? At table? TV on?	Food/Drink description & preparation	Brand Name	Portion size or quantity _eaten_
		How to describe what you had and how much you had can be found on pages 16 - 21		
		6am to 9am		
8.00 am	Café take away – eating on my way to work Alone	Cappuccino, no sugar	Starbucks	Medium size
		Blueberry muffin, regular not low fat	Starbucks	One
8.45 am	Office desk Alone No TV Not at table	Tap water		300 ml glass
		9am to 12 noon		
10 am	Office desk Alone No TV Not at table	Banana		One, medium size
		Black tea semi-skimmed milk, no sugar	Typhoo Asda	Large Mug A lot

Time	Where? With Whom? At table? TV on?	Food/Drink description & preparation	Brand Name	Portion size or quantity eaten
		12 noon to 2pm		
1 pm	Work tea room With colleague No TV At table	Crayfish sandwich multiseed bread, wholemeal, medium cut, crayfish in lemon mayonnaise, no other spread rocket leaves	M&S pre-packed Sandwich	2 slices Medium filling 6 to 8
		Apple & Raspberry fruit drink	J2O	1 bottle, 275ml
		2pm to 5pm		
4.30 pm	Friends House Lounge With Friend Not at table TV on	Coffee, instant Semi-skimmed milk Fairy Cake, homemade, see recipe	Kenco	Medium mug A lot 1 cake

Time slot	Where? With Whom? At table? TV on?	Food/Drink description & preparation	Brand Name	Portion size or quantity eaten
		5pm to 8pm		
7.30 pm	Kitchen/Diner With boyfriend At table No TV	Chicken in creamy mushroom and white wine sauce for 2, oven	Sainsbury's, 370g (wrapper collected)	½ pack
		White rice, boiled	Easy cook, Italian, Sainsbury's	2C
		Wine 13% alcohol	Sauvignon Blanc, New Zealand	1 small glass, 125ml
		8pm to 10pm		
9.15 pm	Sitting Room With boyfriend Not at table TV on	Squash, apple & blackcurrant, no added sugar,	Sainsbury's	1 average glass, 200ml
		Crisps	Pringles, sour cream and chives	5
		10pm to 6am		
11.30 pm	Bedroom Alone Not at table TV on	Water	tap	1 medium glass

Was the amount of **food** that you had today about what you usually have, less than usual, or more than usual?

Yes, usual ☐

No, **less** than usual ☑

No, **more** than usual ☐

Please tell us why you had less than usual

Felt unwell

Please tell us why you had more than usual

Was the amount you had to **drink** today, including water, tea, coffee and soft drinks [and alcohol], about what you usually have, less than usual, or more than usual?

Yes, usual ☐

No, **less** than usual ☑

No, **more** than usual ☐

Please tell us why you had less than usual

Felt unwell

Please tell us why you had more than usual

Did you **finish all the food and drink** that you recorded in the diary today?

Yes ✓   No ☐

If no, please **go back to the diary and make a note of any leftovers**

Did you take any **vitamins, minerals or other food supplements** today?

Yes ✓   No ☐

If yes, **please describe the supplements you took below**

Brand	Name (in full) including strength	Number of pills, capsules, teaspoons
Holland & Barrett	Evening Primrose Oil – 1000mg	1 capsule
Holland & Barrett	Super EPA fish oil – 1000mg	1 capsule

Please record over the page details of any recipes or (if not already described) ingredients of made up dishes or take-away dishes.

Write in recipes or ingredients of made up dishes or take-away dishes

NAME OF DISH: *Fairy Cakes*

SERVES: *makes 20 cakes*

Ingredients	Amount	Ingredients	Amount
Tate & Lyle caster sugar	175g	Silver Spoon icing sugar	140g
Anchor butter, unsalted	175g	Yellow food colouring	3 drops
eggs	3	water	2 tablespoons
Homepride self-raising flour	175g		
Baking powder	1 teaspoon		

Brief description of cooking method

Mix together and bake for 15 min.

Mix icing sugar with water and add colouring. Approx. 1 teaspoon of icing on each cake

Spoon size does matter!!! When describing amounts check the spoons you use with the life size pictures at the back of this diary

Food/Drink	Description & Preparation	Portion size or quantity
Bacon	Back, middle, streaky; smoked or un-smoked; fat eaten; dry-fried or fried in oil/fat (type used) or grilled rashers	Number of rashers
Baked beans	Standard, reduced salt or reduced sugar	Spoons, weight of tin
Beefburger (hamburger)	Home-made (ingredients), from a packet or take-away; fried (type of oil/fat), microwaved or grilled; economy; with or without bread roll, with or without salad e.g. lettuce, tomato	Large or small, ounces or in grams if info on package
Beer	What sort e.g. stout, bitter, lager; draught, canned, bottled; % alcohol or low-alcohol or home-made	Number of pints or half pints, size of can or bottle
Biscuits	What sort e.g. cheese, wafer, crispbread, sweet, chocolate (fully or half coated), shortbread, home-made	Number, size (standard or mini variety)
Bread (see also sandwiches)	Wholemeal, granary, white or brown; currant, fruit, malt; large or small loaf; sliced or unsliced loaf	Number of slices; thick, medium or thin slices
Bread rolls	Wholemeal, white or brown; alone or with filling; crusty or soft	Size, number of rolls
Breakfast cereal (see also porridge)	What sort e.g. Kellogg's cornflakes; any added fruit and/or nuts; Muesli – with added fruit, no added sugar/salt variety	Spoons or picture 1
Buns and pastries	What sort e.g. iced, currant or plain, jam, custard, fruit, cream; type of pastry; homemade or bought	Size, number
Butter, margarine & fat spreads	Give full product name	Thick/average/thin spread; spoons
Cake	What sort: fruit (rich), sponge, fresh cream, iced, chocolate coated; type of filling e.g. buttercream, jam	Individual or size of slice, packet weight, picture 10

Spoon size does matter!!! When describing amounts check the spoons you use with the life size pictures at the back of this diary

Food/Drink	Description & Preparation	Portion size or quantity
Cereal bars	What sort; with fruit/nuts, coated with chocolate/yoghurt; fortified with vitamins/minerals	Weight/size of bar; from multipack
Cheese	Type e.g. cheddar, cream, cottage, soft; low fat	Picture 9, or number of slices, number of spoons
Chips	Fresh, frozen, oven, microwave, take-away (where from); thick/straight/crinkle/fine cut; type of oil/fat used for cooking	Picture 4, as A, B, or C or 2 x B, etc
Chocolate(s)	What sort e.g. plain, milk, white, fancy, diabetic; type of filling;	Weight/size of bar
Coffee	With milk (see section on milk); half milk/half water; all milk; ground/filter, instant; decaffeinated. If café/takeaway, was it cappuccino, latte etc	Cups or mugs, size of takeaway e.g. small. medium
Cook-in sauces	What sort; pasta, Indian, Chinese, Mexican; tomato, white or cheese based; does meat or veg come in sauce; jar or can	Spoons, size of can or jar
Cream	Single, whipped, double or clotted; dairy or non-dairy; low-fat; fresh, UHT/Longlife; imitation cream e.g. Elmlea	Spoons
Crisps	What sort e.g. potato, corn, wheat, maize, vegetable etc; low-fat or low-salt; premium variety e.g. Kettle chips, Walker's Sensations	Packet weight, standard or from multipack
Custard	Pouring custard or egg custard; made with powder and milk/sugar, instant, ready to serve (tinned or carton); low fat, sugar free	Spoons
Egg	Boiled, poached, fried, scrambled, omelette (with or without filling); type of oil/fat, milk added	Number of eggs, large, medium or small
Fish (including canned)	What sort e.g. cod, tuna; fried (type of oil/fat), grilled, poached (water or milk) or steamed; with batter or breadcrumbs; canned in oil, brine or tomato sauce	Size of can or spoons (for canned fish) or picture 7 for battered fish

Spoon size does matter!!!! When describing amounts check the spoons you use with the life size pictures at the back of this diary

Food/Drink	Description & Preparation	Portion size or quantity
Fish cakes & fish fingers	Type of fish; plain or battered or in breadcrumbs; fried, grilled, baked or microwaved; economy	Size, number, packet weight
Fruit - fresh	What sort; eaten with or without skin	Small, medium or large
Fruit - stewed/canned	What sort; sweetened or unsweetened; in fruit juice or syrup; juice or syrup eaten	Spoons, weight of can
Fruit – juice (pure)	What sort e.g. apple, orange; sweetened or unsweetened; pasteurised or UHT/Longlife; freshly squeezed; added vitamins/minerals, omega 3	Glass (size or volume) or carton size
Ice cream	Flavour; dairy or non-dairy alternatives e.g. soya; luxury/premium	Spoons/ scoops
Jam, honey	What sort; low-sugar/diabetic; shop bought/brand or homemade	Spoons, heaped or level, or thin or thick spread
Marmalade	Type; low-sugar; thick cut; shop bought/brand or homemade	Spoons, heaped or level, or thin or thick spread
Meat (see also bacon, burgers & sausages)	What sort; cut of meat e.g. chop, breast, minced; lean or fatty; fat removed or eaten; skin removed or eaten; how cooked; with or without gravy	Large/small/medium, spoons, or picture 6 for stew portion
Milk	What sort; whole, semi-skimmed, skimmed or 1% fat; fresh, sterilized, UHT, dried; soya milk (sweetened/unsweetened), goats' milk, rice milk, oat milk; flavoured; fortified with added vitamins and/or minerals	Pints, glass (size or volume) or cup. On cereal: *damp/normal/ drowned*. In tea/coffee: *a little/some/a lot*

Spoon size does matter!!!! When describing amounts check the spoons you use with the life size pictures at the back of this diary

Food/Drink	Description & Preparation	Portion size or quantity
Nuts	What sort; dry roasted, ordinary salted, honey roasted; unsalted	Packet weight, handful
Pie (sweet or savoury)	What sort/filling; one pastry crust or two; type of pastry	Individual or slice, or picture 8
Pizza	Thin base/deep pan or French bread; topping e.g. meat, fish, veg; stuffed crust	Individual, slice, fraction of large pizza e.g. ¼
Porridge	Made with oats or cornmeal or instant oat cereal; made with milk and/or water; added sugar, honey, syrup or salt; with milk or cream	Bowls, spoons
Potatoes (see also chips)	Old or new; baked, boiled, roast (type of oil/fat); skin eaten; mashed (with butter/spread and with or without milk); fried/chips (type of oil/fat); instant; any additions e.g. butter	Mash – spoons, number of half or whole potatoes, small or large potatoes
Pudding	What sort; e.g. steamed sponge; with fruit; mousse; instant desserts; milk puddings	Spoons, picture 10 for slice of sponge
Rice	What sort; e.g. basmati, easy cook, long or short grain; white or brown; boiled or fried (type of oil/fat)	Spoons or picture 2
Salad	Ingredients; if with dressing what sort (oil and vinegar, mayonnaise)	Amount of each component
Sandwiches and rolls	Type of bread/roll (see Bread & Rolls); butter or margarine; type of filling; including salad, mayonnaise, pickle etc. If shop-bought, where from?	Number of rolls or slices of bread; amount of butter/margarine (on both slices?); amount of filling
Sauce – cold (including mayonnaise)	Tomato ketchup, brown sauce, soy sauce, salad cream, mayonnaise; low fat;	Spoons

Spoon size does matter!!!! When describing amounts check the spoons you use with the life size pictures at the back of this diary

Food/Drink	Description & Preparation	Portion size or quantity
Sauce – hot (see also cook-in sauces)	What sort; savoury or sweet; thick or thin; for gravy - made with granules, stock cube, dripping or meat juices	Spoons
Sausages	What sort; e.g. beef, pork; fried (type of oil/fat) or grilled; low fat	Large or small, number
Sausage rolls	Type of pastry	Size - jumbo, standard, mini
Scone	Fruit, sweet, plain, cheese; type of flour; homemade	Small, medium or large
Savoury snacks - in packet	What sort: e.g. Cheddars, cheese straws, Twiglets, Pretzels	Size (standard or mini variety), packet weight
Smoothies	If homemade give recipe. If shop-bought, what does it contain e.g. fruit, milk/yoghurt, fruit juice	Glass or bottle (size or volume)
Soft drinks – squash/ concentrate/cordial	Flavour; no added sugar/low calorie/sugar free; "high" juice; fortified with added vitamins and/or minerals	Glass (size or volume)
Soft drinks – carbonated/fizzy	Flavour; diet/low-calorie; canned or bottled; cola – caffeine free	Glass, can or bottle (size or volume)
Soft drinks – ready to drink	Flavour; no added sugar/low calorie/sugar free; real fruit juice? If so, how much?; fortified with added vitamins and/or minerals	Glass, carton or bottle (size or volume)
Soup	What sort; cream or clear; fresh/chilled, canned, instant or vending machine. If home-made, give recipe	Spoons, bowl or mug
Spaghetti, other pasta	What sort; fresh/chilled or dried; white, wholemeal; canned in sauce; type of filling if ravioli, cannelloni etc	Spoons (or how much dry pasta) or picture 3

Spoon size does matter!!!! When describing amounts check the spoons you use with the life size pictures at the back of this diary

Food/Drink	Description & Preparation	Portion size or quantity
Spirits	What sort: e.g. whisky, gin, vodka, rum	Measures as in pub
Sugar	Added to cereals, tea, coffee, fruit, etc; what sort; e.g. white, brown, demerara	Heaped or level teaspoons
Sweets	What sort: e.g. toffees, boiled sweets, diabetic, sugar-free	Number, packet weight
Tea	With/without milk (see section on milk); decaffeinated, herb	Mugs or cups
Vegetables (not including potatoes)	What sort; how cooked/raw; additions e.g. butter, other fat or sauce	Spoons, number of florets or sprouts, weight from tins or packet
Wine, sherry, port	White, red; sweet, dry; % alcohol or low-alcohol	Glass (size or volume)
Yoghurt (inc drinking yoghurt), fromage frais	What sort: e.g. natural/plain or flavoured; creamy, Greek, low-fat, very low fat/diet, soya; with fruit pieces or fruit flavoured; twinpot; fortified with added vitamins and/or minerals; longlife/UHT; probiotic	Pot size or spoons
Home-made dishes	Please say what the dish is called (record recipe or details of dish if you can in the section provided) and how many persons it serves	Spoons – heaped or level, number, size
Ready-made meals	Full description of product; does it contain any accompaniments e.g. rice, vegetables, sauces; chilled or frozen; microwaved, oven cooked, boil-in-the-bag; low fat, healthy eating range. Enclose label and ingredients list if possible in your plastic bag	Packet weight (if didn't eat whole packet describe portion consumed)
Take-away food or food eaten out	Please say what the dish is called and give main ingredients if you can. Give name of a chain restaurant e.g. McDonalds	Spoons, portion size e.g. small/medium/large

Use the pictures to help you indicate the size of the portion you have eaten.
Write on the food record the picture number and size A, B or C nearest to your own helping.

Remember that the pictures are much smaller than life size.
The actual size of the dinner plate is 10 inches (25cm), the side plate, 7 inches (18cm), and the bowl, 6.3 inches (16cm).

The tables on pages 16-21 also give examples of foods that you might eat and how much information is required about them.

1. Breakfast cereals

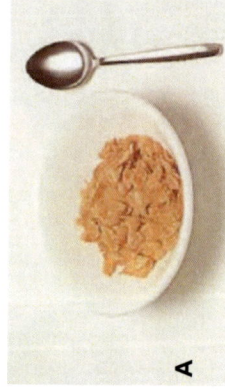

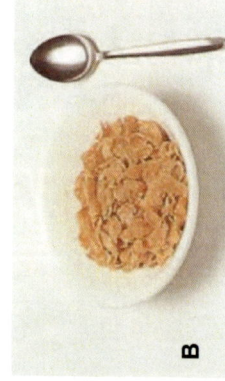

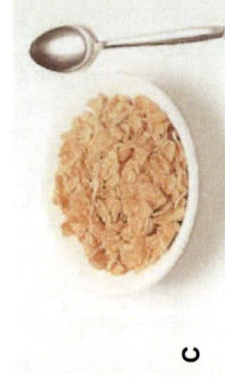

A   B   C

2. Rice

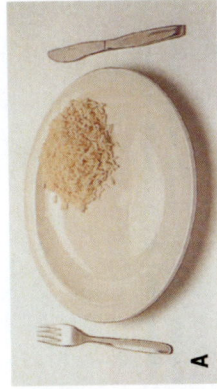 A

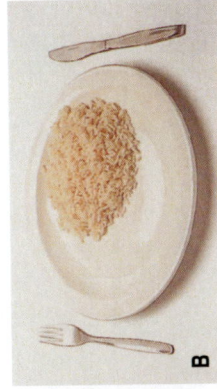 B

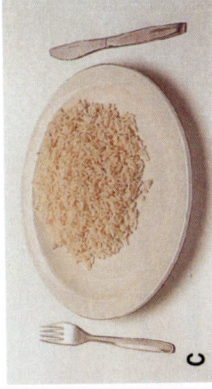 C

3. Spaghetti

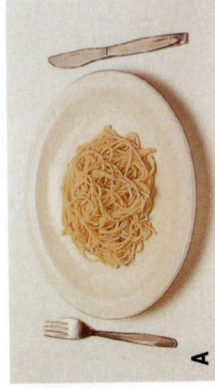 A

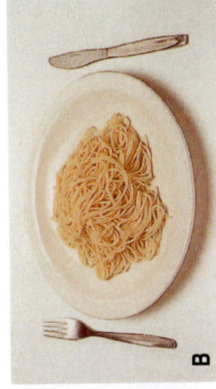 B

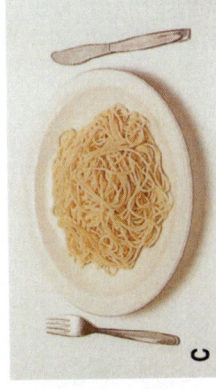 C

4. Chips

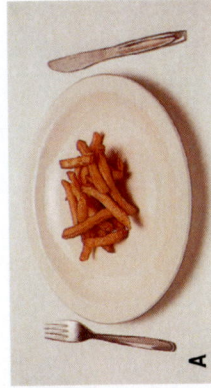 A

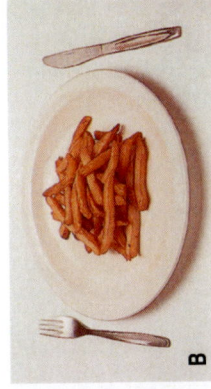 B

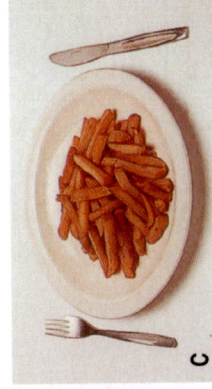 C

5. Broccoli/ cauliflower

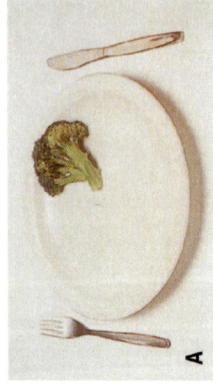

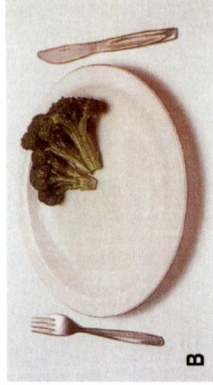

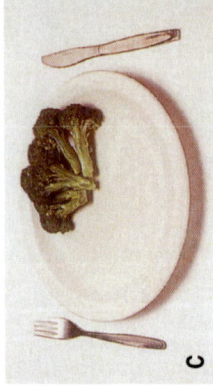

6. Stew /curry

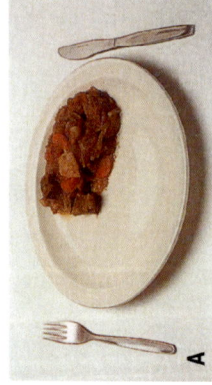

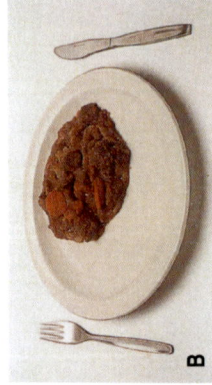

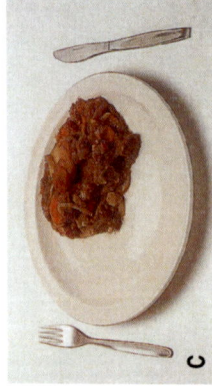

7. Battered fish

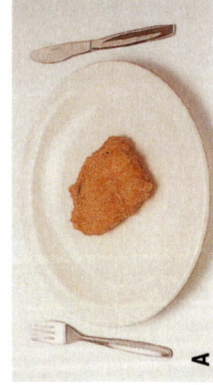

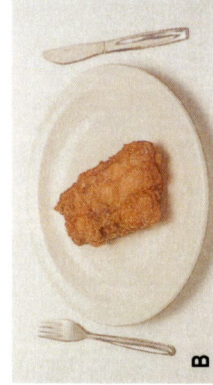

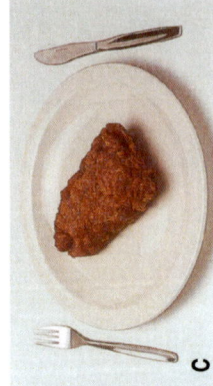

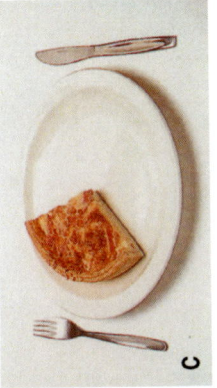

C

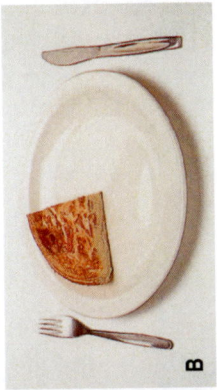

B

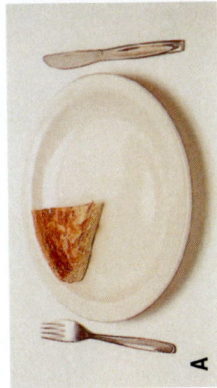

A

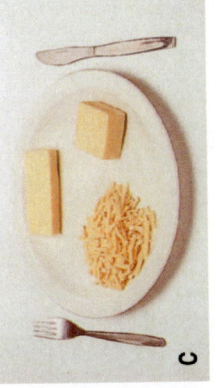

C

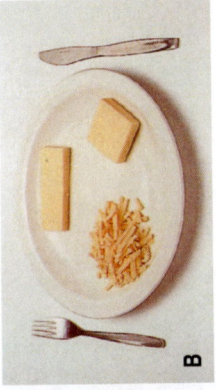

B

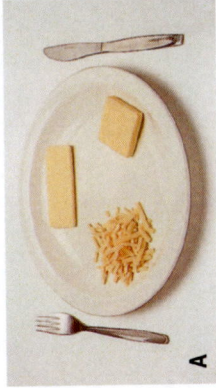

A

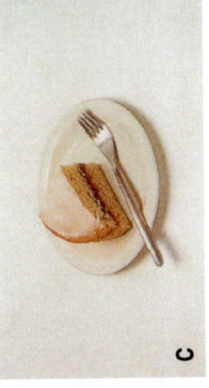

C

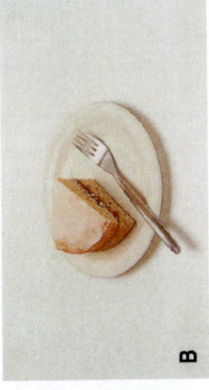

B

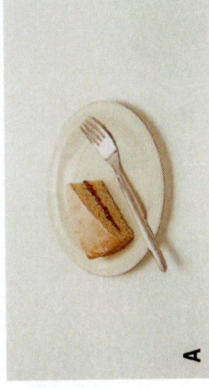

A

8. Quiche / Pie

9. Cheese

10. Sponge cake

Typical quantities of drinks in various containers measured in millilitres (ml)

	Small glass	Average glass	Large glass	Vending cup	Cup	Mug
Soft drinks	150	200	300			
Wine	125	175	250			
Hot drinks				170	190	260

Glasses come in different shapes and sized. On the next page is a life size glass showing approximate volumes. You can use this picture as a guide for estimating how much volume of drink the glass holds you are drinking from.

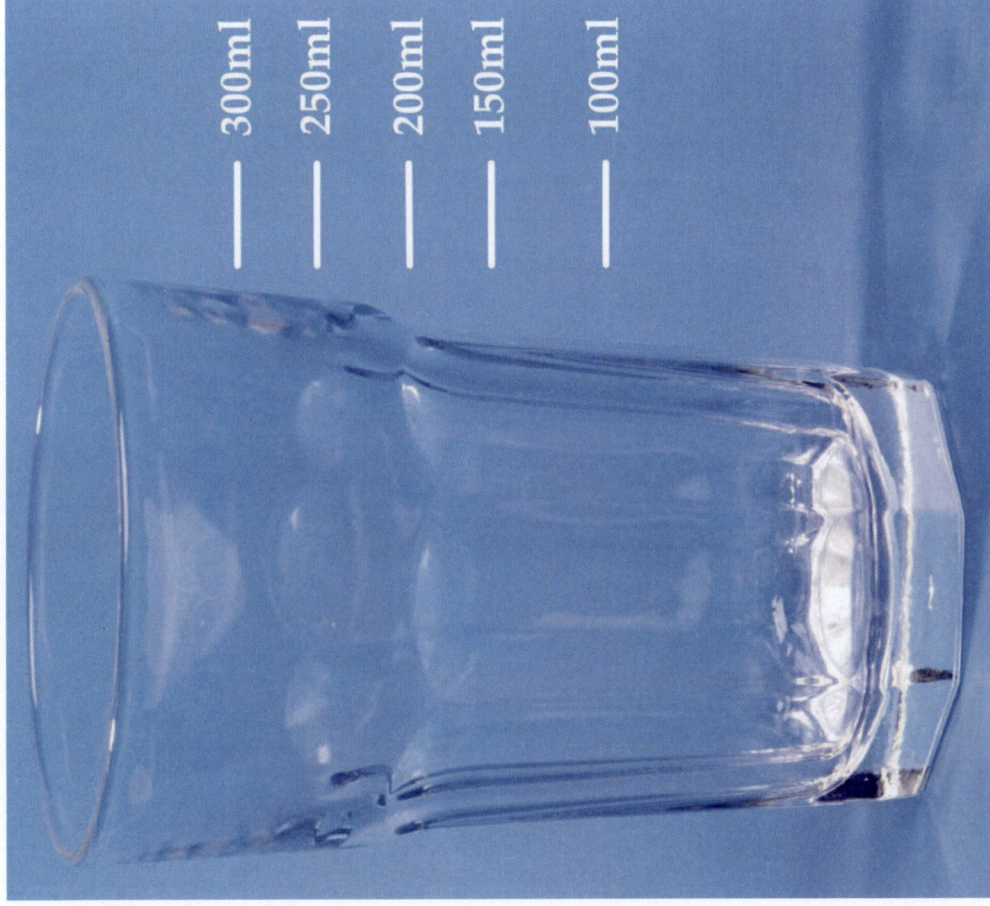

300ml

250ml

200ml

150ml

100ml

Life Size Glass

DAY 1

Day 1:		Date:		
Time	Where? With Whom? TV on? At table?	Food/Drink description & preparation	Brand Name	Portion size or quantity _eaten_
		How to describe what you had and how much you had can be found on pages 16 – 21		
		6am to 9am		
		9am to 12 noon		

Time	Where? With Whom? TV on? At table?	Food/Drink description & preparation	Brand Name	Portion size or quantity eaten
12 noon to 2pm				
2pm to 5pm				

Time	Where? With Whom? TV on? At table?	Food/Drink description & preparation	Brand Name	Portion size or quantity eaten
5pm to 8pm				
8pm to 10pm				
10pm to 6am				

Was the amount of **food** that you had today about what you usually have, less than usual, or more than usual?

Yes, usual ☐   No, **less** than usual ☐   No, **more** than usual ☐

Please tell us why you had less than usual

Please tell us why you had more than usual

Was the amount you had to **drink** today, including water, tea, coffee and soft drinks [and alcohol], about what you usually have, less than usual, or more than usual?

Yes, usual ☐   No, **less** than usual ☐   No, **more** than usual ☐

Please tell us why you had less than usual

Please tell us why you had more than usual

Did you **finish all the food and drink** that you recorded in the diary today?

Yes ☐   No ☐

If no, please **go back to the diary and make a note of any leftovers**

Did you take any **vitamins, minerals or other food supplements** today?

Yes ☐   No ☐

If yes, **please describe the supplements you took below**

Brand	Name (in full) including strength	Number of pills, capsules, teaspoons

Please record on the next pages details of any recipes or (if not already described) ingredients of made up dishes or take-away dishes.

Write in recipes or ingredients of made up dishes or take-away dishes

NAME OF DISH:

Serves:

Ingredients	Amount	Ingredients	Amount

Brief description of cooking method

Write in recipes or ingredients of made up dishes or take-away dishes

NAME OF DISH:

Serves:

Ingredients	Amount	Ingredients	Amount

Brief description of cooking method

DAY 2

Day 2:		Date:		
Time	Where? With Whom? TV on? At table?	Food/Drink description & preparation	Brand Name	Portion size or quantity eaten
		How to describe what you had and how much you had can be found on pages 16 - 21		
		6am to 9am		
		9am to 12 noon		

Time	Where? With Whom? TV on? At table?	Food/Drink description & preparation	Brand Name	Portion size or quantity <u>eaten</u>
12 noon to 2pm				
2pm to 5pm				

Time	Where? With Whom? TV on? At table?	Food/Drink description & preparation	Brand Name	Portion size or quantity eaten
5pm to 8pm				
8pm to 10pm				
10pm to 6am				

Was the amount of **food** that you had today about what you usually have, less than usual, or more than usual?

| Yes, usual | No, **less** than usual | No, **more** than usual |

Please tell us why you had less than usual

Please tell us why you had more than usual

Was the amount you had to **drink** today, including water, tea, coffee and soft drinks [and alcohol], about what you usually have, less than usual, or more than usual?

| Yes, usual | No, **less** than usual | No, **more** than usual |

Please tell us why you had less than usual

Please tell us why you had more than usual

Did you **finish all the food and drink** that you recorded in the diary today?

Yes ☐   No ☐

If no, please **go back to the diary and make a note of any leftovers**

Did you take any **vitamins, minerals or other food supplements** today?

Yes ☐   No ☐

If yes, **please describe the supplements you took below**

Brand	Name (in full) including strength	Number of pills, capsules, teaspoons

Please record on the next pages details of any recipes or (if not already described) ingredients of made up dishes or take-away dishes.

Write in recipes or ingredients of made up dishes or take-away dishes

NAME OF DISH:

Serves:

Ingredients	Amount	Ingredients	Amount

Brief description of cooking method

Write in recipes or ingredients of made up dishes or take-away dishes

NAME OF DISH:

Serves:

Ingredients	Amount	Ingredients	Amount

Brief description of cooking method

DAY 3

Day 3:		Date:		
Time	Where? With Whom? TV on? At table?	Food/Drink description & preparation	Brand Name	Portion size or quantity eaten
		How to describe what you had and how much you had can be found on pages 16 - 21		
6am to 9am				
9am to 12 noon				

Time	Where? With Whom? TV on? At table?	Food/Drink description & preparation	Brand Name	Portion size or quantity eaten
12 noon to 2pm				
2pm to 5pm				

Time	Where? With Whom? TV on? At table?	Food/Drink description & preparation	Brand Name	Portion size or quantity eaten
5pm to 8pm				
8pm to 10pm				
10pm to 6am				

Was the amount of **food** that you had today about what you usually have, less than usual, or more than usual?

Yes, usual ☐   No, **less** than usual ☐   No, **more** than usual ☐

Please tell us why you had less than usual

Please tell us why you had more than usual

Was the amount you had to **drink** today, including water, tea, coffee and soft drinks [and alcohol], about what you usually have, less than usual, or more than usual?

Yes, usual ☐   No, **less** than usual ☐   No, **more** than usual ☐

Please tell us why you had less than usual

Please tell us why you had more than usual

Did you **finish all the food and drink** that you recorded in the diary today?

Yes ☐   No ☐

If no, please **go back to the diary and make a note of any leftovers**

Did you take any **vitamins, minerals or other food supplements** today?

Yes ☐   No ☐

If yes, **please describe the supplements you took below**

Brand	Name (in full) including strength	Number of pills, capsules, teaspoons

Please record on the next pages details of any recipes or (if not already described) ingredients of made up dishes or take-away dishes.

Write in recipes or ingredients of made up dishes or take-away dishes

NAME OF DISH:

Serves:

Ingredients	Amount	Ingredients	Amount

Brief description of cooking method

Write in recipes or ingredients of made up dishes or take-away dishes

NAME OF DISH:

Serves:

Ingredients	Amount	Ingredients	Amount	Ingredients	Amount

Brief description of cooking method

DAY 4

Please remember to complete the general questions on pages 61-66!

Day 4:	Date:			
Time	Where? With Whom? TV on? At table?	Food/Drink description & preparation	Brand Name	Portion size or quantity <u>eaten</u>
		How to describe what you had and how much you had can be found on pages 16 - 21		
6am to 9am				
9am to 12 noon				

Time	Where? With Whom? TV on? At table?	Food/Drink description & preparation	Brand Name	Portion size or quantity eaten
12 noon to 2pm				
2pm to 5pm				

Time	Food/Drink description & preparation	Brand Name	Portion size or quantity _eaten_	Where? With Whom? TV on? At table?
5pm to 8pm				
8pm to 10pm				
10pm to 6am				

Was the amount of **food** that you had today about what you usually have, less than usual, or more than usual?

Yes, usual ☐

No, **less** than usual ☐

No, **more** than usual ☐

Please tell us why you had less than usual

Please tell us why you had more than usual

Was the amount you had to **drink** today, including water, tea, coffee and soft drinks [and alcohol], about what you usually have, less than usual, or more than usual?

Yes, usual ☐

No, **less** than usual ☐

No, **more** than usual ☐

Please tell us why you had less than usual

Please tell us why you had more than usual

Did you **finish all the food and drink** that you recorded in the diary today?

Yes ☐   No ☐

If no, please **go back to the diary and make a note of any leftovers**

Did you take any **vitamins, minerals or other food supplements** today?

Yes ☐   No ☐

If yes, **please describe the supplements you took below**

Brand	Name (in full) including strength	Number of pills, capsules, teaspoons

Please record on the next pages details of any recipes or (if not already described) ingredients of made up dishes or take-away dishes.

Write in recipes or ingredients of made up dishes or take-away dishes

NAME OF DISH:

Serves:

Ingredients	Amount	Ingredients	Amount

Brief description of cooking method

Write in recipes or ingredients of made up dishes or take-away dishes

NAME OF DISH:

Serves:

Ingredients	Amount	Ingredients	Amount

Brief description of cooking method

General questions about your food/ drink during the recording period.

Special diet

1. Did you follow a special diet during the recording period e.g. vegetarian, cholesterol lowering, weight reducing?

Yes ☐

Please specify

No ☐

Milk

2. Which type of milk did you use most often during the recording period?

Whole, fresh, pasteurised ☐

Semi-skimmed fresh, pasteurised ☐

Skimmed (fat free) fresh, pasteurised ☐

1% fat milk, pasteurised ☐

Soya ☐

Type

Dried ☐

Type

Other ☐

Type

Did not use ☐

Tea and coffee

3. How much milk did you usually have in coffee/ tea?

Coffee   A lot ☐   Some ☐   A little ☐   None/did not drink ☐

Tea   A lot ☐   Some ☐   A little ☐   None/did not drink ☐

4. Did you usually sweeten your coffee/ tea with sugar?

Coffee   Yes ☐   How many teaspoons in a mug/cup? ☐   No/did not drink ☐

Tea   Yes ☐   How many teaspoons in a mug/cup? ☐   No/did not drink ☐

5. Did you usually sweeten your coffee/ tea with artificial sweetener?

Coffee   Yes ☐   How many tablets or teaspoons in a mug/cup? ☐   No/did not drink ☐

Tea   Yes ☐   How many tablets or teaspoons in a mug/cup? ☐   No/did not drink ☐

6. Did you drink decaffeinated coffee/ tea during the recording period?

Coffee   Always ☐   Sometimes ☐   Never ☐

Tea   Always ☐   Sometimes ☐   Never ☐

Breakfast cereals

7. How much milk did you usually have on breakfast cereal?

Drowned ☐ Average ☐ Damp ☐ None/did not eat ☐

8. How did you usually make your porridge?

With all water ☐ With all milk ☐ With milk and water ☐ Did not eat ☐

9. Did you usually sweeten or salt your porridge?

With sugar ☐ With honey ☐ With salt ☐ Neither/did not eat ☐

10. How did you usually make your instant oat cereal?

With all water ☐ With all milk ☐ With milk and water ☐ Did not eat ☐

11. Did you usually sweeten or salt your instant oat cereal?

With sugar ☐ With honey ☐ With salt ☐ Neither/did not eat ☐

Fats for spreading and cooking

12. Which type of butter, margarine or other fat spread did you use most often during the recording period? Please record the full product name and fat content

Name:

None ☐

e.g. Flora Omega 3 plus, low fat spread, 38% fat, polyunsaturated

13. How thickly did you spread butter, margarine on bread, crackers etc?

Thick ☐   Medium ☐   Thin ☐   N/A ☐

14. Which type of cooking fat/oil did your household use most often over the recording period? Please record the full product name e.g. *Sainsbury's sunflower oil*

Name:

None ☐

Bread

15. Which type of bread did you eat most often during the recording period?

White ☐   Granary ☐   Wholemeal ☐   Brown ☐

50/50 bread e.g. Hovis Best of Both ☐   Other ☐   *Type*   Did not eat ☐

16. Was it a large loaf or a small loaf?

Large ☐   Small ☐

17. If the bread was shop bought, how was it sliced?

Thick ☐   Medium ☐   Thin ☐   Unsliced ☐   N/A ☐

Meat

18. If you ate meat during the recording period, did you eat the visible fat?

Always ☐   Sometimes ☐   Never ☐   Did not eat meat ☐

19. If you ate poultry (e.g. chicken, turkey) during the recording period, did you eat the skin?

Always ☐   Sometimes ☐   Never ☐   Did not eat poultry ☐

Fruit and vegetables

20. If you ate apples during the recording period, did you eat the skin?

Always ☐   Sometimes ☐   Never ☐   Did not eat ☐

21. If you ate pears during the recording period, did you eat the skin?

Always ☐   Sometimes ☐   Never ☐   Did not eat ☐

22. If you ate new potatoes during the recording period, did you eat the skin?

Always ☐   Sometimes ☐   Never ☐   Did not eat ☐

23. If you ate baked/jacket potatoes during the recording period, did you eat the skin?

Always ☐   Sometimes ☐   Never ☐   Did not eat ☐

Salt

24. Do you add salt to your food at the table?

Always ☐   Sometimes ☐   Never ☐

25. Do you add salt substitute to your food at the table? *e.g. LoSalt*

Always ☐   Sometimes ☐   Never ☐

Water

26. Which type of water did you drink most often during the recording period?

Tap ☐   Filtered ☐   Bottled ☐ *brand* _____   Did not drink ☐

Thank you for completing this diary.

Acknowledgements

Thanks for permission to use pictures from:

Nelson, M., Atkinson, M.
& Meyer, J. (1997).
A Photographic Atlas of Food Portion Sizes.
London, MAFF Publications.

NATIONAL DIET AND NUTRITION SURVEY

Food and Drink Diary *Instructions*

NDNS (I) Diary_Instructions_A5, April 09 REC Ref. 07/H0604/113

For use from 01/04/10

NATIONAL DIET AND NUTRITION SURVEY

Food and Drink Diary Instructions

If you have any queries about how to complete the diary please contact a member of the NDNS Team at NatCen on freephone **0800 652 4572** between 8.30am-5.30pm.

PLEASE READ THROUGH THESE PAGES BEFORE STARTING YOUR DIARY

We would like you to keep this diary of <u>everything you eat and drink</u> over 4 days. Please include all food consumed at home and outside the home e.g. work, college or restaurants. It is very important that you do not change what you normally eat and drink just because you are keeping this record. Please keep to your usual food habits.

<u>Day and Date</u>
Please write down the day and date at the top of the page each time you start a new day of recording.

<u>Time Slots</u>
Please note the time of each eating occasion into the space provided.

<u>Where and with whom?</u>
For each eating occasion, please tell us what **room or part of the house** you were in when you ate, e.g. kitchen, living room, If you ate at your work canteen, a restaurant, fast food chain or your car, write that location down. We would also like to know **who you share your meals with**, e.g. whether you ate alone or with others. If you ate with others please describe their relationship to you e.g. partner, children, colleagues, or friends. We would also like to know **when you ate at a table** and **when you were watching television whilst eating**. For those occasions where you were **not** at a table or watching TV please write 'Not at table' or 'No TV' rather than leaving it blank.

<u>What do you eat?</u>
Please describe the food you eat in as much detail as possible. Be as specific as you can. Pages 28 - 33 will help with the sort of detail we need, like **cooking methods** (fried, grilled, baked etc) and any **additions** (fats, sugar/sweeteners, sauces, pepper etc).

- **Homemade dishes**

  If you have eaten any **homemade dishes** e.g. chicken casserole, please record the name of the recipe, ingredients with amounts (including water or other fluids) for the whole recipe, the number of people the recipe serves, and the cooking method. Write this down in the recipe section at the end of the record day. Record how much of the whole recipe you have eaten in the portion size column (see examples on pages 4 - 27).

- **Take-aways and eating out**

  If you have eaten **take-aways** or **made up dishes not prepared at home** such as at a restaurant or a friend's house, please record as much detail about the ingredients as you can e.g. vegetable curry containing chickpeas, aubergine, onion and tomato.

<u>Brand name</u>
Please note the **brand name** (if known). Most packed foods will list a brand name, e.g. Bird's eye, Hovis, or Supermarket own brands.

- *Labels/Wrappers*

  Labels are an important source of information for us. It helps us a great deal if you enclose, in the plastic bag provided, labels from all **ready meals,** labels from **foods of lesser known brands** and also from any **supplements** you take.

Portion sizes

Examples for how to describe the **quantity** or **portion size** you had of a particular food or drink are shown on pages 28 - 33.

For foods, quantity can be described using:
- **household measures**, e.g. 1 teaspoon (tsp) of sugar, 2 thick slices of bread, 4 tablespoons (tbsp) of peas, ½ cup of gravy. Be careful when describing amounts in spoons that you are referring to the correct spoon size. Compare the spoons you use with the life size pictures at the back of this diary.
- **weights from labels**, e.g. 4oz steak, 420g tin of baked beans, 125g pot of yoghurt
- **number of items**, e.g. 4 fish fingers, 2 pieces of chicken nuggets, 1 regular size jam filled doughnut
- **picture examples** for specific foods on pages 34 - 36.

For drinks, quantity can be described using:
- the **size of glass, cup etc** (e.g. large glass) or the **volume** (e.g. 300ml). Examples of typical drinks containers are on 38 – 39.
- **volumes from labels** (e.g. 330ml can of fizzy drink).

We would like to know the **amount that was actually eaten** which means taking **leftovers** into account. You can do this in two ways:
1. Record what was served and note what was not eaten e.g. 3 tbsp of peas, only 2 tbsp eaten; 1 large sausage roll, ate only ½
2. Only record the amount actually eaten i.e. 2 tbsp of peas; ½ a large sausage roll

Was it a typical day?

After each day of recording you will be prompted to tell us whether this was a typical day or whether there were any reasons why you ate and drank more or less than usual.

Supplements

At the end of each recording day there is a section for providing information about any supplements you took. Brand name, full name of supplement, strength and the amount taken should be recorded.

When to fill in the diary

Please record your eating as you go, not from memory at the end of the day. Use written notes on a pad if you forget to take your diary with you. Each diary day covers a 24hr period, so please include any food or drinks that you may have had during the night. Remember to include foods and drinks between meals (snacks) including water.

Overleaf you can see examples of 4 days that have been filled in by different people. These examples show you how we would like you to record your food and drink, for example a ready meal and a homemade dish.

It only takes a few minutes for each eating occasion!

Thank you for your time – we really appreciate it!

Day: *Thurs* **Date:** *31 March*

Time	Where? With whom? TV on? Table?	Food/Drink description & preparation	Brand Name	Portion size or quantity <u>eaten</u>
		How to describe what you had and how much you had can be found on pages 28-34		
		6am to 9am		
6.30 am	*Kitchen* *Alone* *No TV* *Not at table*	*Filter coffee, decaffeinated* *milk (fresh, semi-skimmed)* *Sugar white*	*Douwe Egberts* *Silverspoon*	*Mug* *A little* *1 level tsp*
7.30 am	*Kitchen* *Partner* *TV on* *At table*	*Filter coffee with milk and sugar* *Cornflakes* *Milk (fresh, semi-skimmed)* *Toast, granary medium sliced* *Light spread* *Marmalade*	*As above* *Tesco's own* *Hovis* *Flora* *Hartleys*	*As above* *1B* *drowned* *1 slice* *med spread* *1 heaped tsp*
		9am to 12 noon		
10.15 am	*Office desk* *Alone* *No TV* *Not at table*	*Instant coffee, not decaffeinated* *Milk (fresh, whole)* *Sugar brown*	*Kenco*	*Mug* *A little* *1 level tsp*
11 am	*Office desk* *Alone* *No TV* *Not at table*	*Digestive biscuit – chocolate coated on one site*	*McVities*	*2*

Time	Where? With whom? TV on? Table?	Food/Drink description & preparation	Brand Name	Portion size or quantity _eaten_
		12 noon to 2pm		
12.30 pm	Work tea room With colleagues No TV At table	Ham salad sandwich from home Bread, wholemeal, thick sliced Light spread	Tesco's own Flora	2 slices thin spread on 1 slice
		Low fat Mayonnaise Smoked ham thinly sliced Lettuce, iceberg Cucumber with skin	Hellmans Tesco's own	2 teaspoons 2 slices 1 leaf 4 thin slices
		Unsweetened orange juice from canteen	Tropicana	250ml carton
		Apple with skin from home, Braeburn		medium size, core left
		2pm to 5pm		
3 pm	Meeting room With supervisor No TV Not at table	Tea, decaffeinated Milk (fresh, whole) Jaffa cake – mini variety	Twinings Tesco's own McVities	Mug Some 6

Time	Where? With whom? TV on? Table?	Food/Drink description & preparation	Brand Name	Portion size or quantity eaten
		5pm to 8pm		
6.30 pm	Pub, partner No TV At table	Gin Tonic water diet Lager 3.8% alcohol Salted peanuts	Gordon's Schweppes Draught, Carlsberg KP	Single measure 1/2 small glass 1 pint 1 handful
8 pm	Dining room Family No TV At table	Spaghetti, wholemeal Bolognese sauce (see recipe) Courgettes (fried in butter) Tinned peaches in juice (juice drained) Single cream UHT Orange squash No Added Sugar	Tesco's own Prince's Sainsbury's own	3b 6 tablespoons 4 tablespoons 3 halves 1 tablespoon 200ml glass, 1 part squash, 3 parts tap water
		8pm to 10pm		
9 pm	Sitting room Alone TV on Not at table	Grapes, green, seedless Chocolates, chocolate creams Potato crisps, Prawn Cocktail	Bendicks Walkers	15 2 25g bag from multipack
		10pm to 6am		
10.30 pm	Bed room Partner No TV Not at table	Camomile tea (no milk or sugar)	Twinings	1 mug

Was the amount of **food** that you had today about what you usually have, less than usual, or more than usual?

Yes, usual [ ] No, **less** than usual [✓] No, **more** than usual [ ]

Please tell us why you had less than usual

Please tell us why you had more than usual

Was the amount you had to **drink** today, including water, tea, coffee and soft drinks [and alcohol], about what you usually have, less than usual, or more than usual?

Yes, usual [ ] No, **less** than usual [ ] No, **more** than usual [✓]

Please tell us why you had less than usual

Please tell us why you had more than usual

Went to pub after work

Did you **finish all the food and drink** that you recorded in the diary today?

Yes ✓   No ☐

If no, please **go back to the diary and make a note of any leftovers**

Did you take any **vitamins, minerals or other food supplements** today?

Yes ✓   No ☐

If yes, **please describe the supplements you took below**

Brand	Name (in full) including strength	Number of pills, capsules, teaspoons
Healthspan	Omega3 fish oil with vitamin A, C, D & E	2 capsules
Boots	Calcium (1000mg) with vitamin D	1 tablet
Holland & Barrett	Vitamin C 60mg	1 tablet

Please record over the page details of any recipes or (if not already described) ingredients of made up dishes or take-away dishes.

Write in recipes or ingredients of made up dishes or take-away dishes

NAME OF DISH: Bolognese sauce

SERVES: 4

Ingredients	Amount	Ingredients	Amount
Co-op low fat beef mince	500g	Lea & Perrins worcester sauce	dash
garlic	3 cloves		
onion	1 medium		
sweet red pepper	1 medium		
Napoli chopped tomatoes	400g tin		
Tesco tomato puree	1 tablespoon		
Tesco olive oil	1 tablespoon		
mixed herbs	1 dessertspoon		

Brief description of cooking method

Fry onion & garlic in oil, add mince and fry till brown.

Add pepper, tomatoes, puree, Worcester sauce & herbs. Simmer for 30 mins

Day:	Friday	Date: 28.09.2007		
Time	**Where?** **With whom?** **TV on?** **Table?**	**Food/Drink description & preparation**	**Brand Name**	**Portion size or quantity eaten**
	How to describe what you had and how much you had can be found on pages 28-34			
		6am to 9am		
8.00 am	Café take away – eating on my way to work Alone	Cappuccino, no sugar Blueberry muffin, regular not low fat	Starbucks Starbucks	Medium size One
8.45 am	Office desk Alone No TV Not at table	Tap water		300 ml glass
		9am to 12 noon		
10am	Office desk Alone No TV Not at table	Banana Black tea semi-skimmed milk, no sugar	 Typhoo Asda	One, medium size Large Mug A lot

Time	Where? With whom? TV on? Table?	Food/Drink description & preparation	Brand Name	Portion size or quantity eaten
		12 noon to 2pm		
1 pm	Work tea room With colleague No TV At table	Crayfish sandwich multiseed bread, medium cut, crayfish in lemon mayonnaise, no other spread rocket leaves	M&S pre-packed Sandwich	2 slices Medium filling 6 to 8
		Apple & Raspberry fruit drink	J2O	1 bottle, 275ml
		2pm to 5pm		
4.30 pm	Friends House Lounge With Friend Not at table TV on	Coffee, instant Semi-skimmed milk	Kenco	Medium mug A lot
		Fairy Cake, homemade, see recipe		1cake

Time	Where? With whom? TV on? Table?	Food/Drink description & preparation	Brand Name	Portion size or quantity eaten
		5pm to 8pm		
7.30 pm	Kitchen/Diner With boyfriend At table No TV	Chicken in creamy mushroom and white wine sauce for 2, oven	Sainsbury's, 370g (wrapper collected)	½ pack
		White rice (homemade), boiled	Easy cook, Italian, Sainsbury's	1C
		Wine 13% alcohol	Sauvignon Blanc, New Zealand	1 small glass, 125ml
		8pm to 10pm		
9.15 pm	Sitting Room With boyfriend Not at table TV on	Squash, apple & blackcurrant, no added sugar,	Sainsbury's	1 average glass, 200ml
		Crisps	Pringles, sour cream and chives	5
		10pm to 6am		
11.30 pm	Bedroom Alone Not at table TV on	Water	tap	1 medium glass

Was the amount of **food** that you had today about what you usually have, less than usual, or more than usual?

| Yes, usual | ☐ | No, **less** than usual | ✓ | No, **more** than usual | ☐ |

Please tell us why you had less than usual

Felt unwell

Please tell us why you had more than usual

Was the amount you had to **drink** today, including water, tea, coffee and soft drinks [and alcohol], about what you usually have, less than usual, or more than usual?

| Yes, usual | ☐ | No, **less** than usual | ✓ | No, **more** than usual | ☐ |

Please tell us why you had less than usual

Felt unwell

Please tell us why you had more than usual

Did you **finish all the food and drink** that you recorded in the diary today?

Yes [✓]   No [ ]

If no, please **go back to the diary and make a note of any leftovers**

Did you take any **vitamins, minerals or other food supplements** today?

Yes [✓]   No [ ]

If yes, **please describe the supplements you took below**

Brand	Name (in full) including strength	Number of pills, capsules, teaspoons
Holland & Barrett	Evening Primrose Oil – 1000mg	1 capsule
Holland & Barrett	Super EPA fish oil – 1000mg	1 capsule

Please record over the page details of any recipes or (if not already described) ingredients of made up dishes or take-away dishes.

Write in recipes or ingredients of made up dishes or take-away dishes

NAME OF DISH: *Fairy Cakes* **SERVES:** *makes 20 cakes*

Ingredients	Amount	Ingredients	Amount
Tate & Lyle caster sugar	175g	Silver Spoon icing sugar	140g
Anchor butter, unsalted	175g	Yellow food colouring	3 drops
Eggs from market	3	water	2 tablespoons
Homepride self-raising flour	175g		
Baking powder	1 teaspoon		

Brief description of cooking method

Mix together and bake for 15 min.

Mix icing sugar with water and add colouring. Approx. 1 teaspoon of icing on each cake

Day: Monday | **Date:** 11 June 20007

How to describe what you had and how much you had can be found on pages 28-34

Time	Where? With whom? TV on? Table?	Food/Drink description & preparation	Brand Name	Portion size or quantity eaten
		6am to 9am		
7am	Dining Room Wife TV on At table	Porridge Made with semi-skimmed milk Honey	Quaker Sainsburys Sainsburys	30g sachet 200ml milk 2 tsp
		Orange Juice, 100% juice	Tropicana	1/4 pint
		9am to 12 noon		
10am	Work desk Colleagues No TV Not at table	Coffee, white, with sugar (bean to cup)	Vending machine	Regular size vending cup
		Bourbon biscuits	Tesco's	2 biscuits

Time	Where? With whom? TV on? Table?	Food/Drink description & preparation	Brand	Portion size or quantity eaten
		12 noon to 2pm		
1pm	Work Restaurant Colleagues At table No TV	Pepperoni pizza with peppers and olives – thin crust	Made in work restaurant	9 inch, ate 1/3
		Salad – Tomatoes Cucumber Lettuce (iceberg) Carrots		4 cherry About 6 slices About 4 leaves About 10 slices
		Thousand Island Dressing	Tesco	1 tbsp
		Coca-cola, standard		330ml can
		2pm to 5pm		
3pm	Work desk Alone No TV Not at table	Bottle of water Banana	Evian	500ml bottle 1 large

Time	Where? With whom? TV on? Table?	Food/Drink description & preparation	Brand	Portion size or quantity eaten
5pm to 8pm				
7pm	Indian Restaurant Wife and Friends No TV At table	Papadum		1 and half
		Mango Chutney		About 4 teasp
		Cucumber Raita		About 4 teasp
		Chicken Tikka		1 chicken breast
		Prawn Bhuna		3 serving spoons
		Niramish (Vegetable side dish, including okra, tomato)		1/2 of dish (about 4 table spoons)
		Pilau Rice		1 dish
		Keema Nan		1/2 of a large size nan
		Onion Bhaji		1 large bhaji
		Beer 4.6% alcohol	Corona	3 bottles
		Water	Don't know	2 med glasses
8pm to 10pm				
9pm	Pub Wife and Friends TV on At table	Beer, draught, 3.8% alcohol	Carlsberg	2 pints
		Salt and Vinegar Crisps, Crinkle cut	McCoys	1 handful
10pm to 6am				

Was the amount of **food** that you had today about what you usually have, less than usual, or more than usual?

Yes, usual ✓

No, **less** than usual ☐

No, **more** than usual ☐

Please tell us why you had less than usual

Please tell us why you had more than usual

Was the amount you had to **drink** today, including water, tea, coffee and soft drinks [and alcohol], about what you usually have, less than usual, or more than usual?

Yes, usual ☐

No, **less** than usual ☐

No, **more** than usual ✓

Please tell us why you had less than usual

Please tell us why you had more than usual

More beer than usual as celebrating birthday

Did you **finish all the food and drink** that you recorded in the diary today?

Yes ☑   No ☐

If no, please **go back to the diary and make a note of any leftovers**

Did you take any **vitamins, minerals or other food supplements** today?

Yes ☐   No ☑

If yes, **please describe the supplements you took below**

Brand	Name (in full) including strength	Number of pills, capsules, teaspoons

Please record over the page details of any recipes or (if not already described) ingredients of made up dishes or take-away dishes.

Write in recipes or ingredients of made up dishes or take-away dishes

NAME OF DISH:

SERVES:

Ingredients	Amount	Ingredients	Amount

Brief description of cooking method

Day: Friday **Date:** 7 Sept 2007

Time	Where? With whom? TV on? Table?	Food/Drink description & preparation	Brand	Portion size or quantity eaten
		How to describe what you had and how much you had can be found on pages 28-34		
		6am to 9am		
7.30 am	Dining room Friends No TV At table	Cooked breakfast: Pork sausages, fried in sunflower oil	Walls	2 regular size
		Unsmoked streaky bacon, grilled, fat eaten	Tesco	2 rashers
		Mushrooms, fried		6
		Baked beans	Heinz	2 tbsp
		Hash browns, oven baked	Birds Eye	2
		Tomato, grilled		1, medium
		Orange juice	Tropicana	Small glass
		Tea	Twinings	1 mug
		Whole milk	Sainsbury's	Dash
		White Sugar	Silverspoon	2 heaped teasp
		9am to 12 noon		
10am	Work desk Alone No TV Not at table	White coffee, no sugar	Vending machine	1 cup

Time	Where? With whom? TV on? Table?	Food/Drink description & preparation	Brand	Portion size or quantity eaten
		12 noon to 2pm		
1pm	Work canteen Colleagues No TV At table	Soup – minestrone	Don't know	1 soup bowl
		White bread, thick slices from large loaf	Don't know	2 slices
		Butter, salted	Lakeland Dairies	2 portion packs
		2pm to 5pm		
3pm	Work desk Alone No TV Not at table	White coffee	Vending machine	1 cup
		Chocolate digestives (half coated)	McVities	2

Time	Where? With whom? TV on? Table?	Food/Drink description & preparation	Brand	Portion size or quantity eaten
		5pm to 8pm		
8pm	Friend's house Friends (birthday party) Not at table No TV	Buffet: Cheese and tomato pizza Potato salad 4 Sandwiches (all with spread): Tuna, sweetcorn and mayo on white bread Wafer thin ham & cucumber on wholemeal bread Smoked salmon and cream cheese on wholemeal bread Cheddar Cheese and pickle on white bread Quiche Lorraine Water biscuits Cheddar cheese Pickle Beer, 5% alcohol, canned	Don't know Don't know Tesco Carr's Branston's Heineken	1/6 of 9in pizza 1 tbsp See recipe section 1/8 quiche 4 4 thick slices 2 tsp 2 pints
		8pm to 10pm		
9pm	Friend's house Friends TV on Not at table	Beer, 5% alcohol, canned Salted peanuts	Heineken KP	2 pints 2 handfuls
		10pm to 6am		
11pm	Living room Alone TV on Not at table	Dry white wine, 13.5% alcohol	Jacob's Creek	1 small glass

Was the amount of **food** that you had today about what you usually have, less than usual, or more than usual?

Yes, usual ☐

No, **less** than usual ☐

No, **more** than usual ☑

Please tell us why you had less than usual

Please tell us why you had more than usual

Went to party

Was the amount you had to **drink** today, including water, tea, coffee and soft drinks [and alcohol], about what you usually have, less than usual, or more than usual?

Yes, usual ☐

No, **less** than usual ☐

No, **more** than usual ☑

Please tell us why you had less than usual

Please tell us why you had more than usual

Went to party

Did you **finish all the food and drink** that you recorded in the diary today?

Yes [✓]   No [ ]

If no, please **go back to the diary and make a note of any leftovers**

Did you take any **vitamins, minerals or other food supplements** today?

Yes [ ]   No [✓]

If yes, **please describe the supplements you took below**

Brand	Name (in full) including strength	Number of pills, capsules, teaspoons

Please record over the page details of any recipes or (if not already described) ingredients of made up dishes or take-away dishes.

Write in recipes or ingredients of made up dishes or take-away dishes

NAME OF DISH: Buffet sandwiches

SERVES: 1

Ingredients	Amount	Ingredients	Amount
Thick sliced white bread	2 slices	Cheddar cheese	2 slices
Thick sliced wholemeal bread	2 slices	Pickle	2 tsp
Unknown spread	Medium spread on all slices		
Tuna, sweetcorn & Mayo	1 tbsp		
Wafer thin ham	1 slice		
Cucumber	2 slices		
Smoked salmon	1 slice		
Cream cheese	2 tsp		

Brief description of cooking method

Spoon size does matter!!!! When describing amounts check the spoons you use with the life size pictures at the back of this diary

Food/Drink	Description & Preparation	Portion size or quantity
Bacon	Back, middle, streaky; smoked or un-smoked; fat eaten; dry-fried or fried in oil/fat (type used) or grilled rashers	Number of rashers
Baked beans	Standard, reduced salt or reduced sugar	Spoons, weight of tin
Beefburger (hamburger)	Home-made (ingredients), from a packet or take-away; fried (type of oil/fat), microwaved or grilled; economy; with or without bread roll, with or without salad e.g. lettuce, tomato	Large or small, ounces or in grams if info on package
Beer	What sort e.g. stout, bitter, lager; draught, canned, bottled; % alcohol or low-alcohol or home-made	Number of pints or half pints, size of can or bottle
Biscuits	What sort e.g. cheese, wafer, crispbread, sweet, chocolate (fully or half coated), shortbread, home-made	Number, size (standard or mini variety)
Bread (see also sandwiches)	Wholemeal, granary, white or brown; currant, fruit, malt; large or small loaf; sliced or unsliced loaf	Number of slices; thick, medium or thin slices
Bread rolls	Wholemeal, white or brown; alone or with filling; crusty or soft	Size, number of rolls
Breakfast cereal (see also porridge)	What sort e.g. Kellogg's cornflakes; any added fruit and/or nuts; Muesli – with added fruit, no added sugar/salt variety	Spoons or picture 1
Buns and pastries	What sort e.g. iced, currant or plain, jam, custard, fruit, cream; type of pastry; homemade or bought	Size, number
Butter, margarine & fat spreads	Give full product name	Thick/average/thin spread; spoons
Cake	What sort: fruit (rich), sponge, fresh cream, iced, chocolate coated; type of filling e.g. buttercream, jam	Individual or size of slice, packet weight, picture 10

Spoon size does matter!!! When describing amounts check the spoons you use with the life size pictures at the back of this diary

Food/Drink	Description & Preparation	Portion size or quantity
Cereal bars	What sort; with fruit/nuts, coated with chocolate/yoghurt; fortified with vitamins/minerals	Weight/size of bar; from multipack
Cheese	Type e.g. cheddar, cream, cottage, soft; low fat	Picture 9, or number of slices, number of spoons
Chips	Fresh, frozen, oven, microwave, take-away (where from); thick/straight/crinkle/fine cut; type of oil/fat used for cooking	Picture 4, as A, B, or C or 2 x B, etc
Chocolate(s)	What sort e.g. plain, milk, white, fancy, diabetic; type of filling;	Weight/size of bar
Coffee	With milk (see section on milk); half milk/half water; all milk; ground/filter, instant; decaffeinated. If café/takeaway, was it cappuccino, latte etc	Cups or mugs, size of takeaway e.g. small. medium
Cook-in sauces	What sort; pasta, Indian, Chinese, Mexican; tomato, white or cheese based; does meat or veg come in sauce; jar or can	Spoons, size of can or jar
Cream	Single, whipped, double or clotted; dairy or non-dairy; low-fat; fresh, UHT/Longlife; imitation cream e.g. Elmlea	Spoons
Crisps	What sort e.g. potato, corn, wheat, maize, vegetable etc; low-fat or low-salt; premium variety e.g. Kettle chips, Walker's Sensations	Packet weight, standard or from multipack
Custard	Pouring custard or egg custard; made with powder and milk/sugar, instant, ready to serve (tinned or carton); low fat, sugar free	Spoons
Egg	Boiled, poached, fried, scrambled, omelette (with or without filling); type of oil/fat, milk added	Number of eggs, large, medium or small
Fish (including canned)	What sort e.g. cod, tuna; fried (type of oil/fat), grilled, poached (water or milk) or steamed; with batter or breadcrumbs; canned in oil, brine or tomato sauce	Size of can or spoons (for canned fish) or picture 7 for battered fish

Spoon size does matter!!!! When describing amounts check the spoons you use with the life size pictures at the back of this diary

Food/Drink	Description & Preparation	Portion size or quantity
Fish cakes & fish fingers	Type of fish; plain or battered or in breadcrumbs; fried, grilled, baked or microwaved; economy	Size, number, packet weight
Fruit - fresh	What sort; eaten with or without skin	Small, medium or large
Fruit - stewed/canned	What sort; sweetened or unsweetened; in fruit juice or syrup; juice or syrup eaten	Spoons, weight of can
Fruit – juice (pure)	What sort e.g. apple, orange; sweetened or unsweetened; pasteurised or UHT/Longlife; freshly squeezed; added vitamins/minerals, omega 3	Glass (size or volume) or carton size
Hot chocolate, cocoa malted drinks etc	Type; standard/low calorie/lite; instant; all water / half milk half water / all milk (see section on milk); any sugar added	Cup or mug plus how much powder e.g. teaspoons, weight on packet
Ice cream	Flavour; dairy or non-dairy alternatives e.g. soya; luxury/premium	Spoons/ scoops
Jam, honey	What sort; low-sugar/diabetic; shop bought/brand or homemade	Spoons, heaped or level, or thin or thick spread
Marmalade	Type; low-sugar; thick cut; shop bought/brand or homemade	Spoons, heaped or level, or thin or thick spread
Meat (see also bacon, burgers & sausages)	What sort; cut of meat e.g. chop, breast, minced; lean or fatty; fat removed or eaten; skin removed or eaten; how cooked; with or without gravy	Large/small/medium, spoons, or picture 6 for stew portion

Spoon size does matter!!! When describing amounts check the spoons you use with the life size pictures at the back of this diary

Food/Drink	Description & Preparation	Portion size or quantity
Milk	What sort; whole, semi-skimmed, skimmed or 1% fat; fresh, sterilized, UHT, dried; soya milk (sweetened/unsweetened), goats' milk, rice milk, oat milk; flavoured; fortified with added vitamins and/or minerals. Formula milks for toddlers	Pints, glass (size or volume) or cup. On cereal: *damp/normal/drowned*. In tea/coffee: *a little/some/a lot*. Formula: *proportion of formula to water*
Milkshake	Fresh or long life/UHT; dairy or non-dairy alternative e.g. soya; if powder, made up with whole, semi-skimmed, skimmed milk; flavour; fortified with vitamins and/or minerals	Glass (size or volume) cups or volume on bottle/carton
Nuts	What sort; dry roasted, ordinary salted, honey roasted; unsalted	Packet weight, handful
Pie (sweet or savoury)	What sort/filling; one pastry crust or two; type of pastry	Individual or slice, or picture 8
Pizza	Thin base/deep pan or French bread; topping e.g. meat, fish, veg; stuffed crust	Individual, slice, fraction of large pizza e.g. ¼
Porridge	Made with oats or cornmeal or instant oat cereal; made with milk and/or water; added sugar, honey, syrup or salt; with milk or cream	Bowls, spoons
Potatoes (see also chips)	Old or new; baked, boiled, roast (type of oil/fat); skin eaten; mashed (with butter/spread and with or without milk); fried/chips (type of oil/fat); instant; any additions e.g. butter	Mash – spoons, number of half or whole potatoes, small or large potatoes
Pudding	What sort; e.g. steamed sponge; with fruit; mousse; instant desserts; milk puddings	Spoons, picture 10 for slice of sponge
Rice	What sort; e.g. basmati, easy cook, long or short grain; white or brown; boiled or fried (type of oil/fat)	Spoons or picture 2

Spoon size does matter!!!! When describing amounts check the spoons you use with the life size pictures at the back of this diary

Food/Drink	Description & Preparation	Portion size or quantity
Salad	Ingredients; if with dressing what sort (oil and vinegar, mayonnaise)	Amount of each component
Sandwiches and rolls	Type of bread/roll (see Bread & Rolls); butter or margarine; type of filling; including salad, mayonnaise, pickle etc. If shop-bought, where from?	Number of rolls or slices of bread; amount of butter/margarine (on both slices?); amount of filling
Sauce – cold (including mayonnaise)	Tomato ketchup, brown sauce, soy sauce, salad cream, mayonnaise; low fat;	Spoons
Sauce – hot (see also cook-in sauces)	What sort; savoury or sweet; thick or thin; for gravy - made with granules, stock cube, dripping or meat juices	Spoons
Sausages	What sort; e.g. beef, pork; fried (type of oil/fat) or grilled; low fat	Large or small, number
Sausage rolls	Type of pastry	Size - jumbo, standard, mini
Scone	Fruit, sweet, plain, cheese; type of flour; homemade	Small, medium or large
Savoury snacks - in packet	What sort: e.g. Cheddars, cheese straws, Twiglets, Pretzels	Size (standard or mini variety), packet weight
Smoothies	If homemade give recipe. If shop-bought, what does it contain e.g. fruit, milk/yoghurt, fruit juice	Glass or bottle (size or volume)
Soft drinks – squash/ concentrate/cordial	Flavour; no added sugar/low calorie/sugar free; "high" juice; fortified with added vitamins and/or minerals	Glass (size or volume)
Soft drinks – carbonated/fizzy	Flavour; diet/low-calorie; canned or bottled; cola – caffeine free	Glass, can or bottle (size or volume)

Spoon size does matter!!! When describing amounts check the spoons you use with the life size pictures at the back of this diary

Food/Drink	Description & Preparation	Portion size or quantity
Soft drinks – ready to drink	Flavour; no added sugar/low calorie/sugar free; real fruit juice? If so, how much?; fortified with added vitamins and/or minerals	Glass, carton or bottle (size or volume)
Soup	What sort; cream or clear; fresh/chilled, canned, instant or vending machine. If home-made, give recipe	Spoons, bowl or mug
Spaghetti, other pasta	What sort; fresh/chilled or dried; white, wholemeal; canned in sauce; type of filling if ravioli, cannelloni etc	Spoons (or how much dry pasta) or picture 3
Toddler foods	Food in jars: description and ingredients (e.g. vegetable risotto, fruit puree); Dry Foods: description (e.g. baby rice, cauliflower cheese); made up with milk and/or water	Size of jar or packet, spoons for powdered foods (volume of water/milk used to mix with cereal or powder)
Spirits	What sort: e.g. whisky, gin, vodka, rum	Measures as in pub
Sugar	Added to cereals, tea, coffee, fruit, etc; what sort; e.g. white, brown, demerara	Heaped or level teaspoons
Sweets	What sort: e.g. toffees, boiled sweets, diabetic, sugar-free	Number, packet weight
Tea	With/without milk (see section on milk); decaffeinated, herb	Mugs or cups
Vegetables (not including potatoes)	What sort; how cooked/raw; additions e.g. butter, other fat or sauce	Spoons, number of florets or sprouts, weight from tins or packet
Wine, sherry, port	White, red; sweet, dry; % alcohol or low-alcohol	Glass (size or volume)
Yoghurt (inc drinking yoghurt), fromage frais	What sort: e.g. natural/plain or flavoured; creamy, Greek, low-fat, very low fat/diet, soya; with fruit pieces or fruit flavoured; twinpot; fortified with added vitamins and/or minerals; longlife/UHT; probiotic	Pot size or spoons

Spoon size does matter!!!! When describing amounts check the spoons you use with the life size pictures at the back of this diary

Food/Drink	Description & Preparation	Portion size or quantity
Home-made dishes	Please say what the dish is called (record recipe or details of dish if you can in the section provided) and how many persons it serves	Spoons – heaped or level, number, size
Ready-made meals	Full description of product; does it contain any accompaniments e.g. rice, vegetables, sauces; chilled or frozen; microwaved, oven cooked, boil-in-the-bag; low fat, healthy eating range. Enclose label and ingredients list if possible in your plastic bag	Packet weight (if didn't eat whole packet describe portion consumed)
Take-away food or food eaten out	Please say what the dish is called and give main ingredients if you can. Give name of a chain restaurant e.g. McDonalds	Spoons, portion size e.g. small/medium/large

Use the pictures to help you indicate the size of the portion you have eaten.
Write on the food record the picture number and size A, B or C nearest to your own helping.

Remember that the pictures are much smaller than life size.
The actual size of the dinner plate is 10 inches (25cm), the side plate, 7 inches (18cm), and the bowl, 6.3 inches (16cm).

The tables on pages 16-21 also give examples of foods that you might eat and how much information is required about them.

Please note, these photographs should not be used to describe children's portions – please use household measures

1. Breakfast cereals

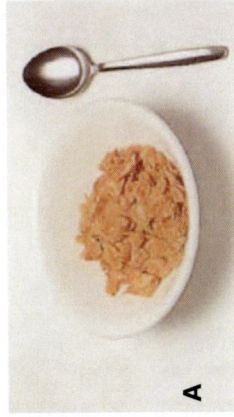

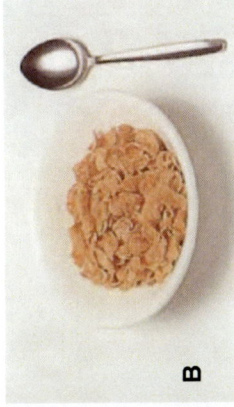

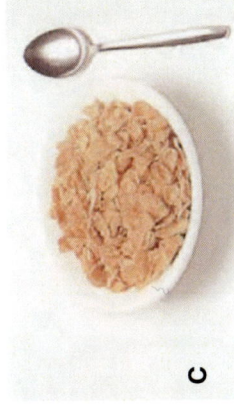

A   B   C

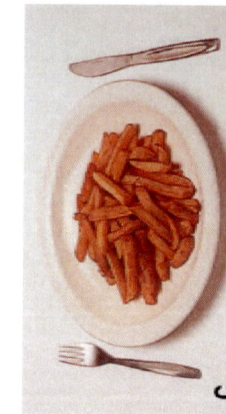

C

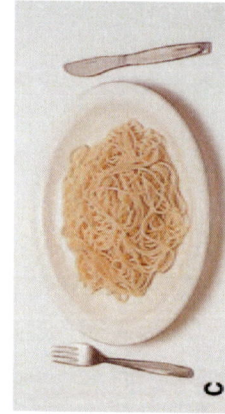

C

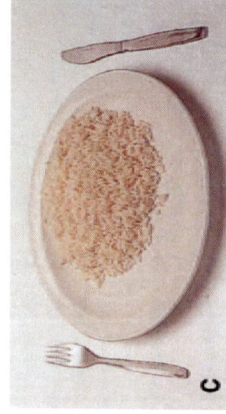

C

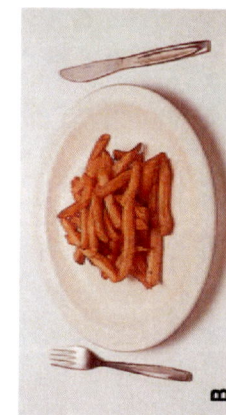

B

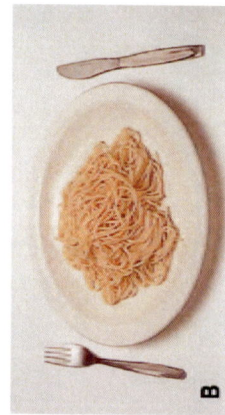

B

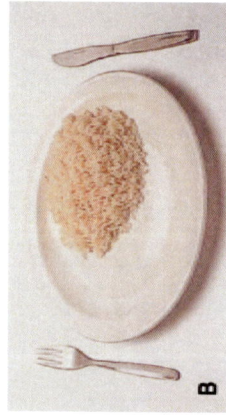

B

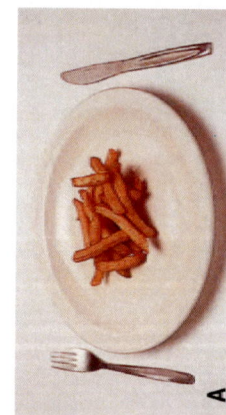

A

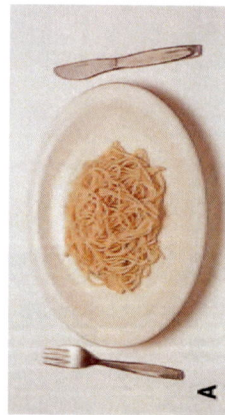

A

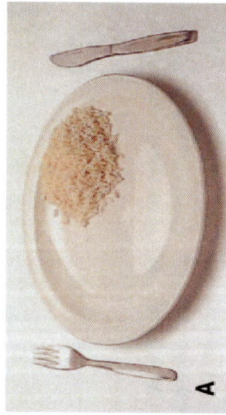

A

2. Rice

3. Spaghetti

4. Chips

5. Broccoli or cauliflower

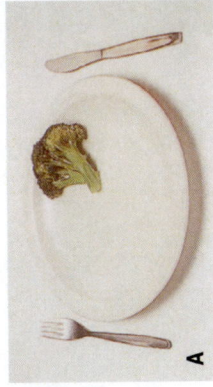

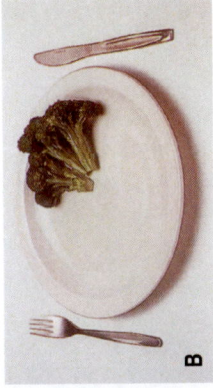

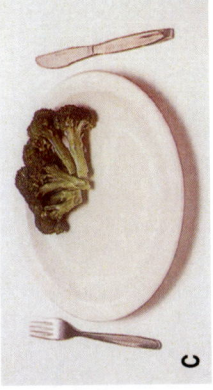

A   B   C

6. Stew or curry

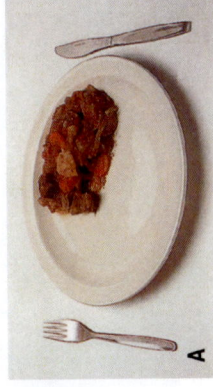

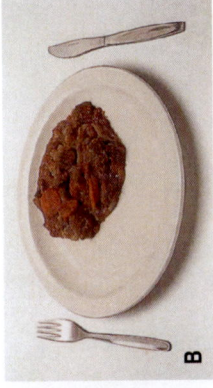

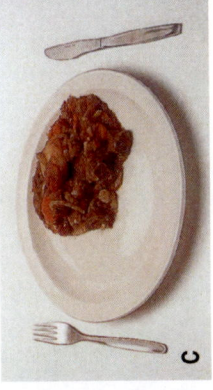

A   B   C

7. Battered fish

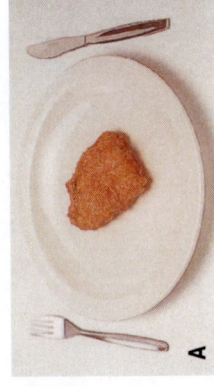

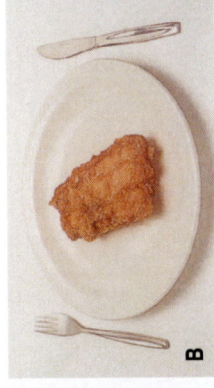

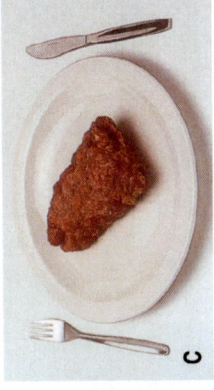

A   B   C

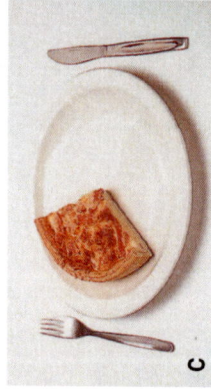

C

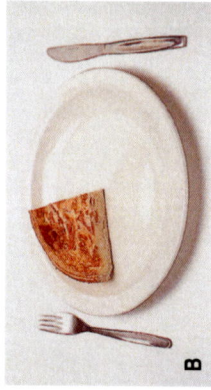

B

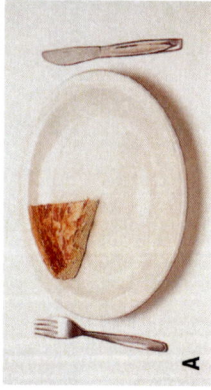

A

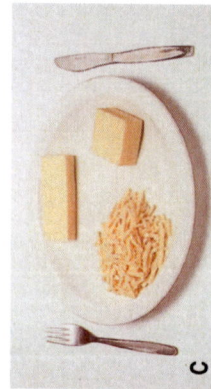

C

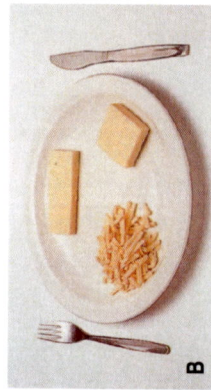

B

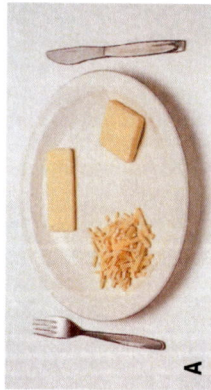

A

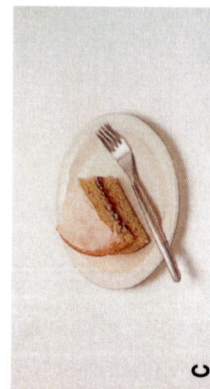

C

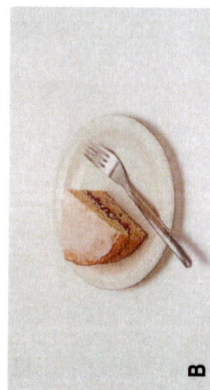

B

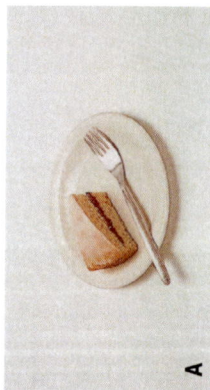

A

8. Quiche / Pie

9. Cheese

10. Sponge cake

Typical quantities of drinks in various containers measured in millilitres (ml)

	Small glass	Average glass	Large glass	Vending cup	Cup	Mug
Soft drinks	150	200	300			
Wine	125	175	250			
Hot drinks				170	190	260

Glasses come in different shapes and sized. On the next page is a life size glass showing approximate volumes. You can use this picture as a guide for estimating how much volume of drink the glass holds you are drinking from.

Life Size Glass

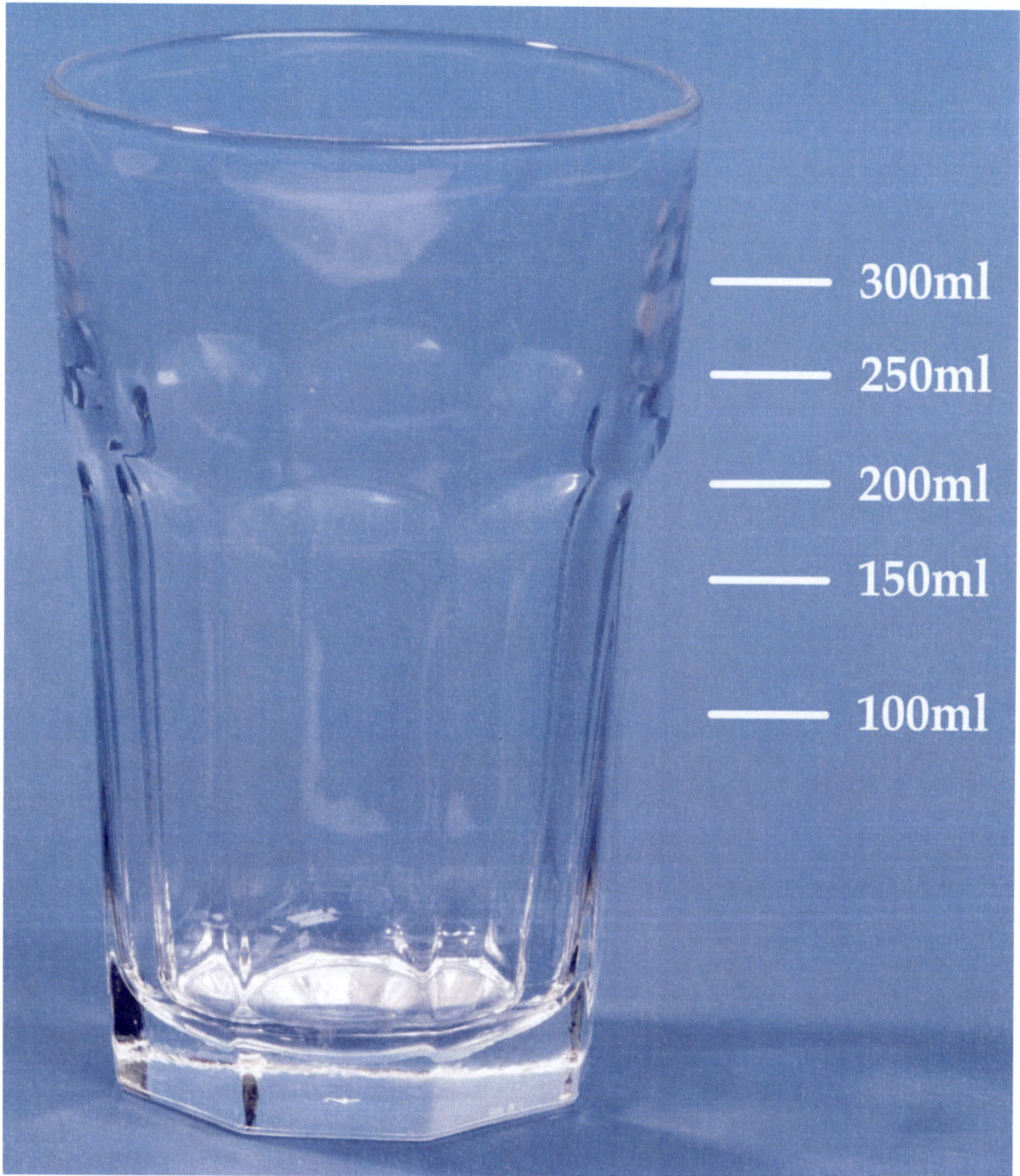

——— 300ml

——— 250ml

——— 200ml

——— 150ml

——— 100ml

Acknowledgements

Thanks for permission to use pictures from:

Nelson, M., Atkinson, M.
& Meyer, J. (1997).
A Photographic Atlas of Food Portion Sizes.
London, MAFF Publications.

NatCen
National Centre *for* Social Research

UCL

MRC | Human Nutrition Research

NATIONAL DIET AND NUTRITION SURVEY

Food and Drink Diary

DIARY START DATE: _____

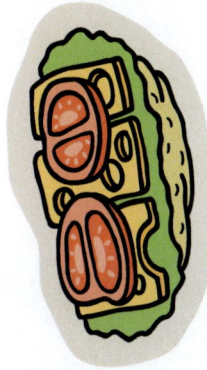

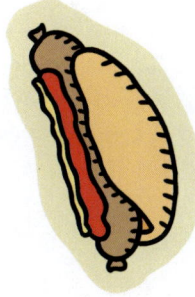

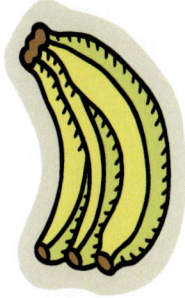

SERIAL NUMBER

CKL   RESPONDENT No

FIRST NAME

Sex: Male / Female

Date of birth:

INTERVIEWER NUMBER:

INTERVIEWER NAME:

NDNS(I) Diary_Child, April 09 REC Ref. 07/H0604/113

For use from 01/04/10

How to fill in your diary

It is very important that you do not change what you normally eat or drink just because you are keeping a diary. Try to write down what you are eating or drinking as soon as you can and not leave it until the end of the day. Record food and drink eaten at home and away from home, such as at school or at a friend's house.

Whenever you have something to eat or drink write down:

When: Each day is divided into time slots from first thing in the morning until late at night until the following morning. Find the appropriate time slot and record the exact time when you eat or drink something in the "time" column.

Where: This could be	Home	Bedroom
	Away	Street, Car/Bus, Café/ Restaurant (specify Mac Donalds, Pizza Hut etc.)
	School	Canteen, Classroom, Playground
With Whom: This could be		Alone
		With family
		With friends

At table: Were you sitting at a table whilst eating or drinking? If yes, record **At table.** If no, record **Not at table.**

Watching TV: Were you watching TV whilst you were eating or drinking? If yes, record **TV on.** If no, record **No TV.**

What:

Describe your food and drink giving as much detail as you can. Include any **extras** like sugar and milk in your tea or cereal, butter or other spreads on your bread and sauces such as ketchup and mayonnaise. **Do not forget to include drinking water.**

If you know how the food was cooked (eg. roast, baked, boiled, fried), please record this. If you're unsure about how the food was cooked, please ask the person who prepared the food if possible.

On pages 12 - 17 you will find help with the sort of detail that is useful.

If you have eaten any **homemade dishes** eg. a stew or sponge cake, please make sure the ingredients and cooking method are recorded in the space provided. You may need to ask the person who prepared the dish to help you with this. If another person at home is also keeping a diary and has recorded the recipes for the same dishes as you in their diary (the ADULT diary), you do NOT need to record these recipes again, just write in your diary "see adult diary". If you have eaten any **take-aways** or any made up dishes not prepared at home such as at a friend's house or in a restaurant, please record as much detail as you can about what was in the dish eg. vegetable curry containing chickpeas, aubergine, onion and tomato.

Brand:

Please make a note of the **brand name** (eg. Heinz, Walkers, Hovis) if you know it. Most packaged foods will list a brand name.

Amount eaten:

You can specify packet (eg. Crisps, Yogurt), or number of individual items (eg. biscuits), or slices (eg. cake, pizza, ham), or teaspoons (eg. sugar), or tablespoons (eg. peas). Be careful when describing amounts in spoons. *Compare the spoon you are using with the life size spoons at the back of this diary so you use the correct name.* You can also write S (small), M (medium) or L (large) portion.

For drinks you can write glass (tell us the size of the glass or volume using page 18 as a guide), cup or mug. You can also write the

weight or volume from the labels on the packaging.

On pages 12 – 18 you will find help with describing how much you had to eat or drink.

We would like to know the **amount that you actually ate,** so you need to think about how much you **leftover.** You can do this in 2 ways:

1. Record how much you were served and then how much you ate e.g. 3 tablespoons of peas, only 2 tablespoons eaten: 1 large sausage roll, ate only half

2. Only record how much you actually ate i.e. 2 tablespoons of peas; half a large sausage roll

Food labels/wrappers:

Please keep the labels or packaging from snacks, sweets, bought sandwiches and ready meals and put them in the plastic bag provided.

Was it a typical day?

After each day of recording you will be prompted to tell us whether this was a usual day (tick yes, usual) or whether there were any reasons why you ate and drank more or less than usual, e.g. I did eat less because I was sick; I drank a lot because I did sports.

Supplements

At the end of each recording day you need to tell us about any supplements you took. If you didn't take any just tick NO. If yes, then please tell us the name of the supplement (e.g. vitamin C), brand (e.g. Boots), strength (it will tell you on the label – e.g. 50 mg) and how many you took (e.g. 1 tablet).

If you have any queries about how to complete the diary please contact a member of the NDNS team on freephone
0800 652 4572 between 8.30am and 5.30pm.

On pages 4-11 of the diary we have filled in a two whole days to show you what to do.

Day EXAMPLE	Day: Thursday	Date: March 31st		
Time	**Where? With whom? TV on? Table?**	**What**	**Brand Name**	**Amount eaten**
		How to describe what you had and how much you had can be found on pages 12-17		
		6am to 9am		
7.30am	Kitchen Family No TV At table	Orange juice, unsweetened, UHT Tea Milk, fresh semi skimmed Sugar white Weetabix Milk as above Sugar as above Toast wholemeal, large loaf Butter unsalted Strawberry Jam	Tesco Tesco Tesco Silverspoon Hovis Anchor Co-op	Large glass Mug A little 2 level teaspoons 2 Drowned 2 heaped teaspoons 2 thin slices thick spread on both 1 teaspoon on one slice
		9am to 12 noon		
11am	School playground With friends	Coca cola diet Potato crisps, Salt and Vinegar	Coca Cola Walkers	330ml can 25g packet from a multipack
12noon	School corridor Alone	Water from water cooler Mars Bar		small plastic cup 1 kingsize
		12 noon to 2pm		
12.45pm	School canteen With friends At table	Sandwich, from home White bread, large loaf Spread Ham unsmoked Cheddar cheese Branston Pickle Apple with skin from home Ribena Light, Ready to Drink, Blackcurrant, from canteen Kitkat from home	Kingsmill Flora Light Tescos	2 med slices thin spread on both slices 1 slice 2 medium slices 1 teaspoon 1 (left core) 220ml carton 2 fingers
1.50pm	School corridor Alone	Chewing gum	Orbit Sugar Free	1 piece

Day EXAMPLE	Day: Thursday	Date: March 31st		
Time	where? with whom? TV on? Table?	what	Brand Name	Amount eaten
2pm to 5pm				
3.45pm	Bus Alone	Wine gums	Maynards	140g packet
4.30pm	Home, sitting room, With family TV on Not at table	Tea (as above) Chocolate Hob Nobs	Mcvitites	mug 3
5pm to 8pm				
6.30pm	Friend's kitchen With friends No TV At table	Chicken in tomato sauce made by friend's mum Tomato fresh Sweetcorn tinned Peach yoghurt low fat Lemon squash No Added Sugar	See recipe Mullerlight Sainsbury's	3 tablespoons 3 slices 1 tablespoon 200g pot medium glass
8pm to 10pm				
8pm	Home, sitting room Alone TV on, Not at table	Satsuma Cream Crackers (no spread)	Jacob's	1 4
9.30pm	Kitchen Alone No TV, At table	Thick cut, frozen chips fried in vegetable oil Brown sauce	HP	small portion 1 dessertspoon
10pm to 6am				
10.30pm	Bedroom Alone TV on Not at table	Hot chocolate drink made with water	Cadbury's	Mug
2am	Bedroom (in bed) Alone No TV	Water tap		½ small glass

Was the amount of **food** that you had today about what you usually have, less than usual, or more than usual?

| Yes, usual ☐ | No, **less** than usual ☐ | No, **more** than usual ☑ |

Please tell us why you had less than usual

Please tell us why you had more than usual

Ate dinner at friend's house

Was the amount you had to **drink** today, including water, tea, coffee and soft drinks [and alcohol], about what you usually have, less than usual, or more than usual?

| Yes, usual ☐ | No, **less** than usual ☑ | No, **more** than usual ☐ |

Please tell us why you had less than usual

Please tell us why you had more than usual

Did you take any vitamin and/or mineral supplements today?   YES ☑   NO ☐

If **YES**, please record details below (and enclose label in plastic bag if possible)

Brand	Name (in full) including strength	Number of pills/capsules/tsps
Bassetts	Soft and chewy vitamins A (800 g), C (60mg), D (5 g) and E (10 mg)	1 pastille
Haliborange	DHA Omega-3 Blackcurrant chewy caps (Each capsule contains 200mg fish oil providing 130mg omega-3)	2 capsules

Did you finish all the food and drink that you recorded in the diary today?

Yes ✓   No ☐

If no, please **go back to the diary and make a note of any leftovers**

Write in recipe or ingredients of made up dishes or take-away dishes

NAME OF DISH: *Chicken in tomato sauce*   **Serves: 4 people**

Ingredients	Amount	Ingredients	Amount
pieces of chicken	3 pieces		
sauce made with tinned tomatoes, green pepper and onions	2 tablespoons		

Brief description of cooking method

Chicken pieces fried in olive oil, then mixed in with tomato and vegetable sauce

How to describe what you had and how much you had can be found on pages 12-17

Day EXAMPLE — Time	Day: Friday Where? With whom? TV on? Table?	Date: April 1st What	Brand Name	Amount eaten
		6am to 9am		
7.45am	Dining Room Family No TV At table	Special K Bliss Strawberry and Chocolate Whole milk Banana Smoothie, made with semi-skimmed milk	Kelloggs Tesco's Homemade see recipe	4 tbsp Drowned 1 medium glass
		9am to 12 noon		
11.30 am	School playground School friends	Orange Juice, unsweetened Mars Bar	Libby's Mars	200ml carton 2 fun size
		12 noon to 2pm		
1pm	School canteen School Friends At table	Roast Chicken Roast Potatoes Boiled Carrots Boiled Peas Gravy Plain sponge pudding with jam Warm chocolate custard		3 slices 2 potatoes 1 tablespoon 1 tablespoon 2 tbsp Small portion 2 dessertspoons

Day EXAMPLE	Day: Friday	Date: April 1st		
Time	Where? With whom? TV on? Table?	What	Brand Name	Amount eaten
		2pm to 5pm		
3.30pm	Car Family	Bottle of water Grapes, green, seedless	Evian	½ bottle – 500mls 10 grapes
4.30pm	Living room Sister TV on Not at table	Ready salted Crisps	Pringles	About 15 crisps
		5pm to 8pm		
7pm	Dining room Family No TV At table	Cheese and tomato pizza, thin base Green beans, boiled Broccoli, boiled Chocolate Mousse, low fat Orange High Juice Squash	Pizza Express (cook at home) Cadburys Robinson's	½ pizza (500g) uncooked 2 tbsp 2 florets 55g pot 1/3 squash & 2/3 water
		8pm to 10pm		
9pm	Bedroom Alone TV on Not at table (in bed)	Semi-skimmed milk	Tesco's	Small glass
		10pm to 6am		

Was the amount of **food** that you had today about what you usually have, less than usual, or more than usual?

Yes, usual	[ ]
No, **less** than usual	[✓]
No, **more** than usual	[ ]

Please tell us why you had less than usual

Felt unwell

Please tell us why you had more than usual

Was the amount you had to **drink** today, including water, tea, coffee and soft drinks [and alcohol], about what you usually have, less than usual, or more than usual?

Yes, usual	[ ]
No, **less** than usual	[✓]
No, **more** than usual	[ ]

Please tell us why you had less than usual

Felt unwell

Please tell us why you had more than usual

Did you take any vitamin and/or mineral supplements today?   YES [ ]   NO [✓]

If **YES**, please record details below (and enclose label in plastic bag if possible)

Brand	Name (in full) including strength	Number of pills/capsules/tsps

Did you **finish all the food and drink** that you recorded in the diary today?

Yes ☑   No ☐

If no, please **go back to the diary and make a note of any leftovers**

Write in recipe or ingredients of made up dishes or take-away dishes

NAME OF DISH: Banana Smoothie   **Serves: 1**

Ingredients	Amount	Ingredients	Amount
Banana	1 small		
Tesco semi-skimmed milk	150ml		
Gales Honey	1 tsp		
Tesco natural unsweetened yogurt	1 tbsp		

Brief description of cooking method

Mix all together with blender

Spoon size does matter!!!! When describing amounts check the spoons you use with the life size pictures at the back of this diary

Food/Drink	Description & Preparation	Amount
Bacon	Back, middle, streaky; smoked or unsmoked; fat eaten; dry-fried or fried in oil/fat (type used) or grilled rashers	Number of rashers
Baked beans	Standard, reduced salt or reduced sugar	Spoons, tin size e.g. 244g
Beefburger (hamburger)	Home-made (ingredients), from a packet or take-away; fried (type of oil/fat), microwaved or grilled; economy; with or without bread roll, with or without salad e.g. lettuce, tomato	Large or small, ounces or in grams if info on package
Biscuits	What sort e.g. cheese, wafer, crispbread, sweet, chocolate (fully or half coated), shortbread, home-made	Number, size (standard or mini variety)
Bread (see also sandwiches)	Wholemeal, granary, white or brown; currant, fruit, malt; large or small loaf; sliced or unsliced loaf	Number of slices; thick, medium or thin slices
Bread rolls	Wholemeal, white or brown; alone or with filling; crusty or soft	Size, number of rolls
Breakfast cereal (see also porridge)	What sort e.g. Kellogg's cornflakes; any added fruit and/or nuts; Muesli – with added fruit, no added sugar/salt variety	Spoons
Buns and pastries	What sort e.g. iced, currant or plain, jam, custard, fruit, cream; type of pastry; homemade or bought	Size, number
Butter, margarine & fat spreads	Give full product name	Thick, average, thin spread on bread/crackers; spoons
Cake	What sort: fruit (rich), sponge, fresh cream, iced, chocolate coated; type of filling e.g. buttercream, jam	Individual or size of slice, packet weight
Cereal bars	What sort; with fruit/nuts, coated with chocolate/yoghurt; fortified with vitamins/minerals	Weight/size of bar; from multipack

Spoon size does matter!!! When describing amounts check the spoons you use with the life size pictures at the back of this diary

Food/Drink	Description & Preparation	Amount
Cheese	Name and type e.g. cheddar, cream, cottage, soft; low fat	Slices, spoons
Chips	Fresh, frozen, oven, microwave, take-away (where from): thick/straight/crinkle/fine cut; type of oil/fat used for cooking	Spoons, portion size, number of chips
Chocolate(s)	What sort e.g. plain, milk, white, fancy, diabetic; type of filling; give brand name	Number, weight/size of bar
Coffee	With milk (see section on milk): half milk/half water; all milk; ground/filter, instant; decaffeinated. If café/takeaway, was it cappuccino, latte etc	Cups or mugs, size of takeaway e.g. small, medium
Cook-in sauces	What sort: pasta, Indian, Chinese, Mexican; tomato, white or cheese based; does meat or veg come in sauce; jar or can	Spoons, size of can or jar
Cream	Single, whipped, double or clotted; dairy or non-dairy; low-fat: fresh, UHT/Longlife; imitation cream e.g. Elmlea	Spoons
Crisps	What sort e.g. potato, corn, wheat, maize, vegetable etc; flavour: low-fat or low-salt; premium variety e.g. Kettle chips; baked variety	Packet weight, standard or from multipack
Custard	Pouring custard or egg custard: made with powder and milk/sugar, instant, ready to serve (tinned or carton): low fat, sugar free	Spoons
Egg	Boiled, poached, fried, scrambled, omelette (with or without filling): type of oil/fat, milk added	Number of eggs, large, medium or small
Fish (including canned)	What sort e.g. cod, tuna, haddock; fried (type of oil/fat), grilled, poached (water or milk) or steamed; with batter or breadcrumbs; canned in oil, brine or tomato sauce	Size of can (e.g. 80g or spoons (for canned fish) or size of fillet
Fish cakes/fish fingers	Type of fish; fried, grilled, baked or microwaved; economy; battered or with coated in breadcrumbs	Size, number
Fruit – fresh	What sort: with or without skin	Small, medium or large

Spoon size does matter!!!! When describing amounts check the spoons you use with the life size pictures at the back of this diary

Food/Drink	Description & Preparation	Amount
Fruit – stewed/canned	What sort; sweetened or unsweetened; in fruit juice or syrup; juice or syrup eaten	Spoons
Fruit – juice (pure)	What sort e.g. apple, orange; sweetened or unsweetened; pasteurised or UHT/Longlife; freshly squeezed	Glass (size or volume) or carton size
Hot chocolate, cocoa malted drinks etc	Type: standard/low calorie/lite; instant; all water / half milk half water / all milk (see section on milk); any sugar added	Cup or mug plus how much powder e.g. teaspoons, weight on packet
Ice cream	Flavour; dairy or non-dairy alternatives e.g. soya; luxury/premium	Spoons/ scoops
Jam, honey	What sort; low-sugar/diabetic; shop bought or homemade	Spoons, heaped or level, or thin or thick spread
Marmalade	What sort; low-sugar; thick cut; shop bought or homemade	Spoons, heaped or level, or thin or thick spread
Meat (see also bacon, burgers & sausages)	What sort; cut of meat e.g. chop, breast, minced; lean or fatty; fat removed or eaten; skin removed or eaten; how cooked; with or without gravy	Large/small/medium, spoons
Milk	What sort; whole, semi-skimmed, skimmed or 1% fat; fresh, sterilized, UHT, dried; soya milk (sweetened/unsweetened), goats' milk, rice milk, oat milk; flavoured; fortified with added vitamins and/or minerals	Pints, glass (size or volume) or cup. On cereal: *damp/normal/drowned.* In tea/coffee: *a little/some/a lot*
Milkshake	Fresh or long life/UHT; dairy or non-dairy alternative e.g. soya; if powder, made up with whole, semi-skimmed, skimmed milk; flavour; fortified with vitamins and/or minerals	Glass (size or volume) cups or volume on bottle/carton
Nuts	What sort; dry roasted, ordinary salted, honey roasted; unsalted	Packet weight, handful
Pie (sweet or savoury)	What sort/filling; one pastry crust or two; type of pastry	Individual or slice

Spoon size does matter!!!! When describing amounts check the spoons you use with the life size pictures at the back of this diary

Food/Drink	Description & Preparation	Amount
Pizza	Thin base/deep pan or French bread; topping e.g. meat, fish, veg; stuffed crust	Individual, slice, fraction of large pizza e.g. $\frac{1}{4}$
Porridge	Made with oats or cornmeal or instant oat cereal; made with milk and/or water; added sugar, honey, syrup or salt; with milk or cream	Spoons or bowl size (small, medium, large)
Potatoes (see also chips)	Old or new; baked, boiled, roast (type of oil/fat); skin eaten; mashed/creamed (with butter, milk etc); fried/chips (type of oil/fat); instant; any additions e.g. butter	Spoons for mash, number of half or whole potatoes
Pudding	What sort; e.g. steamed sponge; with fruit; mousse; instant desserts; milk puddings	Spoons, slices
Rice	What sort; e.g. basmati, easy cook, long or short grain; white or brown; boiled or fried (type of oil/fat)	Spoons
Salad	Ingredients; if with dressing what sort (oil and vinegar, mayonnaise)	Amount of each component: slices, leaves; spoons
Sandwiches and rolls	Type of bread/roll (see Bread & Rolls); butter or margarine; type of filling; including salad, mayonnaise, pickle etc. If shop-bought, where from?	Number of rolls or slices of bread; amount of butter/margarine (on both slices?); amount of filling
Sauce – hot (see also cook-in sauces)	What sort; savoury or sweet; thick or thin; give brand or recipe; for gravy – made with granules, stock cube, dripping or meat juices	Spoons
Sauce – cold (including mayonnaise)	Tomato ketchup, brown sauce, soy sauce, salad cream, mayonnaise; low fat	Spoons
Sausages	What sort; e.g. beef, pork; fried (type of oil/fat) or grilled; low fat; economy	Large or small, number
Sausage rolls	Type of pastry	Number, size e.g. jumbo, standard, mini

Spoon size does matter!!!! When describing amounts check the spoons you use with the life size pictures at the back of this diary

Food/Drink	Description & Preparation	Amount
Scone	Fruit, sweet, plain, cheese; type of flour	Number, size
Savoury snacks – in packet	What sort: e.g. Cheddars, cheese straws, Twiglets, Pretzels	Size (standard or mini variety), packet weight
Smoothies	If homemade give recipe. If shop-bought, what does it contain e.g. fruit, milk/yoghurt, fruit juice	Glass or bottle (size or volume)
Soft drinks – concentrated/squash /cordial	Flavour; no added sugar/low calorie/sugar free; "high" juice; fortified with added vitamins and/or minerals	Glass (size or volume)
Soft drinks – carbonated/fizzy	Flavour; diet/low-calorie; canned or bottled; cola – caffeine free	Glass, can or bottle (size or volume, e.g. 330ml)
Soft drinks – ready to drink	Flavour; no added sugar/low calorie/sugar free; does it contain real fruit juice, if so, how much?; fortified with added vitamins and/or minerals	Glass, carton or bottle (size or volume, e.g. 200ml)
Soup	What sort; cream or clear; fresh/chilled, canned, instant or vending machine. If home-made, give recipe	Spoons, bowl or mug
Spaghetti, other pasta	What sort; fresh or dried; white, wholemeal; boiled, canned in sauce; type of filling if ravioli, cannelloni etc	Spoons
Sugar	Added to cereals, tea, coffee, fruit, etc; what sort; e.g. white, brown, demerara	Heaped or level teaspoons
Sweets	What sort; e.g. toffees, boiled sweets, diabetic, sugar-free	Number, packet weight
Tea	with/without milk (see section on milk); decaffeinated, herb	Mugs or cups

Spoon size does matter!!! When describing amounts check the spoons you use with the life size pictures at the back of this diary

Food/Drink	Description & Preparation	Amount
Vegetables (not including potatoes)	What sort; how cooked or raw; additions e.g. butter, other fat or sauce	Spoons, number of florets or sprouts, weight from tins or packet
Yoghurt (inc drinking yoghurt), fromage frais	What sort: e.g. natural/plain or flavoured; creamy, Greek, low-fat, very low fat/diet, soya; with fruit pieces or fruit flavoured; twinpot; fortified with added vitamins and/or minerals; longlife/UHT; probiotic	Pot size (e.g. 150g) or tablespoons
Home-made dishes	Please say what the dish is called (record recipe or details of dish if you can in the section provided)	Spoons
Ready-made meals	Please give brand name and full description of product; did it contain any accompaniments e.g. rice, vegetables, sauces; chilled or frozen; microwaved, oven cooked, boil-in-the-bag; low fat, healthy eating range. Enclose label and ingredients list if possible in your plastic bag	Packet weight, portion size
Take-away food or food eaten out	Please say what the dish is called and give main ingredients if you can. Give name of a chain restaurant e.g. McDonalds	Spoons, portion size e.g. small/medium/large

Typical quantities of drinks in various containers measured in millilitres (ml)

	Small Glass	Average Glass	Large Glass	Vending Cup	Cup	Mug
Soft Drinks	150	200	300			
Hot Drinks				170	190	260

Here is a life size glass showing what typical quantities look like. You can use this picture as a guide for estimating how much volume of drink the glass holds you are drinking from.

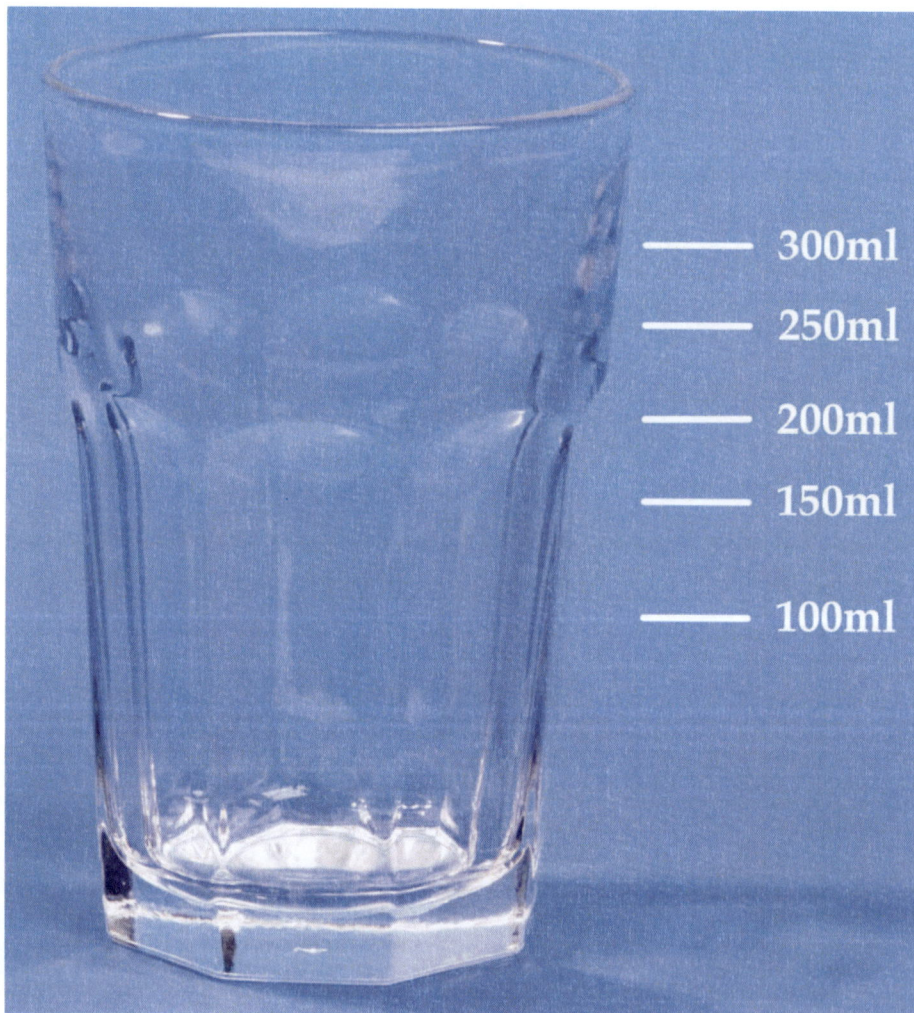

Day 1	Day:	Date:		
Time	where? with whom? TV on? Table?	what	Brand Name	Amount eaten
		How to describe what you had and how much you had can be found on pages 12-17		
		6am to 9am		
		9am to 12 noon		
		12 noon to 2pm		

Day 1	Day:	Date:			
Time	Where? With whom? TV on? Table?	what		Brand Name	Amount eaten
		2pm to 5pm			
		5pm to 8pm			
		8pm to 10pm			
		10pm to 6am			

Was the amount of **food** that you had today about what you usually have, less than usual, or more than usual?

Yes, usual ☐

No, **less** than usual ☐

No, **more** than usual ☐

Please tell us why you had less than usual

Please tell us why you had more than usual

Was the amount you had to **drink** today, including water, tea, coffee and soft drinks [and alcohol], about what you usually have, less than usual, or more than usual?

Yes, usual ☐

No, **less** than usual ☐

No, **more** than usual ☐

Please tell us why you had less than usual

Please tell us why you had more than usual

Did you take any vitamin and/or mineral supplements today?

YES ☐   NO ☐

If **YES**, please record details below (and enclose label in plastic bag if possible)

Brand	Name (in full) including strength	Number of pills/capsules/tsps

Did you finish all the food and drink that you recorded in the diary today?

Yes ☐   No ☐

If no, please go back to the diary and make a note of any leftovers

Write in recipe or ingredients of made up dishes or take-away dishes

NAME OF DISH:		Serves:	
Ingredients	Amount	Ingredients	Amount

Brief description of cooking method

Day 2	Day:	Date:		
Time	where? with whom? TV on? Table?	what	Brand Name	Amount eaten
		How to describe what you had and how much you had can be found on pages 12-17		
6am to 9am				
9am to 12 noon				
12 noon to 2pm				

Day 2	Day:	Date:		
Time	Where? With whom? TV on? Table?	What	Brand Name	Amount eaten
		2pm to 5pm		
		5pm to 8pm		
		8pm to 10pm		
		10pm to 6am		

Was the amount of **food** that you had today about what you usually have, less than usual, or more than usual?

Yes, usual ☐

No, **less** than usual ☐

No, **more** than usual ☐

Please tell us why you had less than usual

Please tell us why you had more than usual

Was the amount you had to **drink** today, including water, tea, coffee and soft drinks [and alcohol], about what you usually have, less than usual, or more than usual?

Yes, usual ☐

No, **less** than usual ☐

No, **more** than usual ☐

Please tell us why you had less than usual

Please tell us why you had more than usual

Did you take any vitamin and/or mineral supplements today?   YES ☐   NO ☐

If **YES**, please record details below (and enclose label in plastic bag if possible)

Brand	Name (in full) including strength	Number of pills/capsules/tsps

Did you finish all the food and drink that you recorded in the diary today?

Yes ☐ No ☐

If no, please **go back** to the diary and **make a note of any leftovers**

Write in recipe or ingredients of made up dishes or take-away dishes

NAME OF DISH:		Serves:		
Ingredients	Amount	Ingredients	Amount	

Brief description of cooking method

Day 3	Day:	Date:		
Time	Where? With whom? TV on? Table?	what	Brand Name	Amount eaten
		How to describe what you had and how much you had can be found on pages 12-17		
6am to 9am				
9am to 12 noon				
12 noon to 2pm				

Day 3	Day:	Date:		
Time	Where? With whom? TV on? Table?	What	Brand Name	Amount eaten
2pm to 5pm				
5pm to 8pm				
8pm to 10pm				
10pm to 6am				

Was the amount of **food** that you had today about what you usually have, less than usual, or more than usual?

Yes, usual ☐

No, **less** than usual ☐

No, **more** than usual ☐

Please tell us why you had less than usual

Please tell us why you had more than usual

Was the amount you had to **drink** today, including water, tea, coffee and soft drinks [and alcohol], about what you usually have, less than usual, or more than usual?

Yes, usual ☐

No, **less** than usual ☐

No, **more** than usual ☐

Please tell us why you had less than usual

Please tell us why you had more than usual

Did you take any vitamin and/or mineral supplements today?

YES ☐   NO ☐

If **YES**, please record details below (and enclose label in plastic bag if possible)

Brand	Name (in full) including strength	Number of pills/capsules/tsps

Did you finish all the food and drink that you recorded in the diary today?

Yes ☐   No ☐

If no, please go back to the diary and make a note of any leftovers

Write in recipe or ingredients of made up dishes or take-away dishes

NAME OF DISH: *Serves:*

Ingredients	Amount	Ingredients	Amount

Brief description of cooking method

Remember to complete the general questions on pages 36-41!

Day 4	Day:	Date:		
Time	Where? With whom? TV on? Table?	what	Brand Name	Amount eaten
		How to describe what you had and how much you had can be found on pages 12-17		
		6am to 9am		
		9am to 12 noon		
		12 noon to 2pm		

Day 4   Day: Date:

Time	Where? With whom? TV on? Table?	What	Brand Name	Amount eaten
2pm to 5pm				
5pm to 8pm				
8pm to 10pm				
10pm to 6am				

Was the amount of **food** that you had today about what you usually have, less than usual, or more than usual?

Yes, usual ☐

No, **less** than usual ☐

No, **more** than usual ☐

Please tell us why you had less than usual

Please tell us why you had more than usual

Was the amount you had to **drink** today, including water, tea, coffee and soft drinks [and alcohol], about what you usually have, less than usual, or more than usual?

Yes, usual ☐

No, **less** than usual ☐

No, **more** than usual ☐

Please tell us why you had less than usual

Please tell us why you had more than usual

Did you take any vitamin and/or mineral supplements today?

YES ☐   NO ☐

If **YES**, please record details below (and enclose label in plastic bag if possible)

Brand	Name (in full) including strength	Number of pills/capsules/tsps

Did you finish all the food and drink that you recorded in the diary today?

Yes ☐   No ☐

If no, please go back to the diary and make a note of any leftovers

Write in recipe or ingredients of made up dishes or take-away dishes

NAME OF DISH:

Serves:

Ingredients	Amount	Ingredients	Amount

Brief description of cooking method

General Questions about your food/ drink during the recording period.

Special diet

1. Did you follow a special diet during the recording period (e.g. vegetarian, weight reducing)?

Yes ☐   No ☐

Please tell us about it

Milk

2. Which type of milk did you use most often during the recording period?

Whole, fresh, pasteurised ☐   Semi-skimmed fresh, pasteurised ☐   Skimmed (fat free) fresh, pasteurised ☐   1% fat milk, fresh pasteurised ☐

Dried ☐   Soya ☐   Did not use ☐

Type

Other ☐

Type

Type

Tea and coffee

3. How much milk did you usually have in coffee/ tea?

	A lot	Some	A little	None/did not drink
Coffee	☐	☐	☐	☐
Tea	☐	☐	☐	☐

4. Did you usually sweeten your coffee/ tea with sugar?

	Yes	How many teaspoons in a mug/cup?	No/did not drink
Coffee	☐	☐	☐
Tea	☐	☐	☐

5. Did you usually sweeten your coffee/ tea with artificial sweetener?

	Yes	How many tablets or teaspoons in a mug/cup?	No/did not drink
Coffee	☐	☐	☐
Tea	☐	☐	☐

6. Did you drink decaffeinated coffee/ tea during the recording period?

	Always	Sometimes	Never
Coffee	☐	☐	☐
Tea	☐	☐	☐

Breakfast cereals

7. How much milk did you usually have on breakfast cereal?

Drowned ☐ Average ☐ Damp ☐ None/did not eat ☐

8. How did you usually make your porridge?

With all water ☐ With all milk ☐ With milk and water ☐ Did not eat ☐

9. Did you usually sweeten or salt your porridge?

With sugar ☐ With honey ☐ With salt ☐ Neither/did not eat ☐

10. How did you usually make your instant oat cereal? e.g. Ready Brek

With all water ☐ With all milk ☐ With milk and water ☐ Did not eat ☐

11. Did you usually sweeten or salt your instant oat cereal?

With sugar ☐ With honey ☐ With salt ☐ Neither/did not eat ☐

Fats for spreading and cooking

12. Which butter, margarine or fat spread did you use most often during the recording period? Please record the full product name and fat content e.g. *Flora Omega 3 plus, low fat spread, 38% fat, polyunsaturated*

Name:

None ☐

13. How thickly did you spread butter, margarine on bread, crackers etc?

Thick ☐   Medium ☐   Thin ☐   None ☐

14. Which cooking fat/oil did your household use most often over the recording period? Please record the full product name. e.g. *Sainsbury's sunflower oil*

Name:

None ☐

Bread

15. Which type of bread did you eat most often during the recording period?

White ☐   Granary ☐   Wholemeal ☐   Brown ☐

50/50 bread e.g. Hovis Best of Both ☐   Other ☐   *Type*

Did not eat ☐

16. Was it a large loaf or a small loaf?

Large ☐   Small ☐

17. If the bread was shop bought, how was it sliced?

Thick ☐   Medium ☐   Thin ☐   Unsliced ☐   N/A ☐

Meat

18. If you ate red meat during the recording period, did you eat the visible fat?

Always ☐   Sometimes ☐   Never ☐   Did not eat meat ☐

19. If you ate poultry (e.g. chicken, turkey) during the recording period, did you eat the skin?

Always ☐   Sometimes ☐   Never ☐   Did not eat poultry ☐

Fruit and vegetables

20. If you ate apples during the recording period, did you eat the skin?

Always ☐   Sometimes ☐   Never ☐   Did not eat ☐

21. If you ate pears during the recording period, did you eat the skin?

Always ☐   Sometimes ☐   Never ☐   Did not eat ☐

22. If you ate new potatoes during the recording period, did you eat the skin?

Always ☐   Sometimes ☐   Never ☐   Did not eat ☐

23. If you ate baked/jacket potatoes during the recording period, did you eat the skin?

Always ☐   Sometimes ☐   Never ☐   Did not eat ☐

Salt

24. Do you add salt to your food at the table?

Always ☐   Sometimes ☐   Never ☐

25. Do you add salt substitute to your food at the table? *e.g. LoSalt*

Always ☐   Sometimes ☐   Never ☐

Cordial/squash/diluting juice

26. Which type of squash/cordial did you drink most often during the recording period?

Ordinary ☐   No added sugar /diet/low calorie ☐   Did not drink ☐

27. Which squash did you use most often during the recording period? Please record the full product name
e.g. Robinsons Peach Fruit & Barley no added sugar

Name: _____

28. How much do you usually dilute your squash (e.g. half squash/half water, or 1 part squash with 4 parts water)?

Please tell us: _____

Water

29. Which type of water did you drink most often during the recording period?

Tap ☐   Filtered ☐   Bottled ☐   brand _____   Did not drink ☐

Thank you for completing this diary.

National Diet and Nutrition Survey

Booklet for 8-12 year olds

In Confidence

Point					Address		CKL	Person no		First name:		

1001-
1005

1006 -
1007

1008

1011

1012 - 1026

Card		Type	Batch		Interviewer no.							Spare
0	1	1										

1009 -
1010

1038

1027 - 1031

1032 - 1037

1039 -
1050

- Here are some questions for you to answer on your own.

- We are interested in your honest answers.

- **We will not tell anyone what your answers are.**

- Look at the instructions on the next page and read what to do.

- Ask the interviewer for help if you do not understand a question or are not sure what to do.

Thank you for taking part in this survey

GREEN

How to answer these questions

- Please read each question carefully

- Most of the questions can be answered by putting a tick in the box
  next to the answer that applies to you, like this

  Yes ☑₁

  No   ☐₂

- Sometimes you have to write a number in the box, for example

  I was **8**₀ years old

  write in

- Next to some of the boxes are arrows and instructions
  They show or tell you which question to answer next.
  If there are no special instructions, just answer the next question.

  No   ☐₂   **Go to question 4**

  Yes ☑₁

  I was **10** years old

  write in

1

Cigarette Smoking

Q1 Have you ever tried smoking a cigarette, even if it was only a puff or two?

Tick one box

1051

No ☐ 2 → **Go to question 2**

Yes ☐ 1

How old were you when you tried smoking a cigarette, even if it was only a puff or two?

1052 - 1053

I was ☐ years old

Write in

Q2 Now read all the following sentences very carefully and tick the box next to the one which best describes you.

Tick one box

1054

I have never smoked ☐ 1 → **Go to question 4**

I have only smoked once or twice ☐ 2

I used to smoke sometimes, but I never smoke a cigarette now ☐ 3

I sometimes smoke, but I don't smoke every week ☐ 4 → **Go to question 3**

I smoke between one and six cigarettes a week ☐ 5

I smoke more than six cigarettes a week ☐ 6

Q3 Did you smoke any cigarettes last week?

Tick one box

1055

No ☐ 2 → **Go to question 4**

Yes ☐ 1

How many cigarettes did you smoke last week?

1056 - 1058

I smoked ☐ cigarettes

Write in

Spare 1059 - 1074

2

Drinking

Q4 Have you ever had a proper alcoholic drink – a whole drink, not just a sip? **Please don't count drinks labelled low alcohol.**

Tick one box
1075

Yes ☐₁ → **Go to question 6**

No ☐₂ → **Go to question 5**

Q5 Have you ever drunk alcopops (such as Bacardi Breezer, Smirnoff Ice, WKD, Reef etc)?

Tick one box
1076

Yes ☐₁ → **Go to question 6**

No ☐₂ → **END**

Q6 How old were you the first time you had a proper alcoholic drink or alcopop?

1077 - 1078

I was ☐ years old

write in

Q7 How often do you usually have an alcoholic drink or alcopop?

Tick one box
1079

Almost every day ☐₁

About twice a week ☐₂

About once a week ☐₃

About once a fortnight ☐₄ → **Go to question 8**

About once a month ☐₅

Only a few times a year ☐₆

I never drink alcohol now ☐₇

3

Q8 When did you **last** have an alcoholic drink or alcopop?

Tick one box
1080

Today [ ] 1

Yesterday [ ] 2

Some other time during the last week [ ] 3

1 week, but less than 2 weeks ago [ ] 4

2 weeks, but less than 4 weeks ago [ ] 5

1 month, but less than 6 months ago [ ] 6

6 months ago or more [ ] 7

Spare 1081 - 1099

Thank you for answering these questions.

Please give the booklet back to the interviewer.

NDNS

National Diet and Nutrition Survey

Booklet for 13-15 year olds

In Confidence

Point					Address		CKL	Person no

1001 -
1005

Address
1006 -
1007

CKL
1008

Person no
1011

First name:
1012 - 1026

Card		Type
0	1	2

1009 -
1010

Type
1038

Batch
1027 - 1031

Interviewer no.
1032 - 1037

Spare
1039 -
1050

- Here are some questions for you to answer on your own.

- We are interested in your honest answers.

- **We will not tell anyone what your answers are**.

- Look at the instructions on the next page and read what to do.

- Ask the interviewer for help if you do not understand a question or are not sure what to do.

Thank you for taking part in this survey

BLUE

How to answer these questions

- Please read each question carefully

- Most of the questions can be answered by putting a tick in the box
  next to the answer that applies to you like this

  Yes ☑ 1

  No   ☐ 2

- Sometimes you have to write a number in the box, for example

  I was **13** . years old

  write in

- Next to some of the boxes are arrows and instructions
  They show or tell you which question to answer next.
  If there are no special instructions, just answer the next question.

  No   ☐ 2 → **Go to Q4**

  Yes ☑ 1

  I was **13** years old

  write in

Cigarette Smoking

Q1 Have you ever tried smoking a cigarette, even if it was only a puff or two?

Tick one box

1051

Yes ☐ 1

No ☐ 2

→ **Go to question 2**

Q2 Now read all the following sentences very carefully and tick the box next to the one which best describes you.

Tick one box

1052

I have never smoked ☐ 1 → **Go to question 5**

I have only smoked once or twice ☐ 2

I used to smoke sometimes, but I never smoke a cigarette now ☐ 3

I sometimes smoke, but I don't smoke every week ☐ 4 → **Go to question 3**

I smoke between one and six cigarettes a week ☐ 5

I smoke more than six cigarettes a week ☐ 6

Q3 How old were you when you tried smoking a cigarette, even if it was only a puff or two?

1053 - 1054

I was ☐ years old → **Go to question 4**

write in

Q4 Did you smoke any cigarettes last week?

Tick one box

1055

No ☐ 2 → **Go to question 5**

Yes ☐ 1

How many cigarettes did you smoke last week?

1056 - 1058

I smoked ☐ cigarettes

Write in Spare 1059 - 1074

Drinking

Q5 Have you ever had a proper alcoholic drink – a whole drink, not just a sip? **Please don't count drinks labelled low alcohol.**

Tick one box

1075

Yes ☐ 1 → **Go to question 7**

No ☐ 2 → **Go to question 6**

Q6 Have you ever drunk alcopops (such as Bacardi Breezer, Smirnoff Ice, WKD, Reef etc)?

Tick one box

1076

Yes ☐ 1 → **Go to question 7**

No ☐ 2 → **END**

Q7 How old were you the first time you had a proper alcoholic drink or an alcopop?

1077 - 1078

I was ☐ years old **Go to question 8**

write in

Q8 How often do you usually have an alcoholic drink or alcopop?

Tick one box

1079

Almost every day ☐ 1

About twice a week ☐ 2

About once a week ☐ 3

About once a fortnight ☐ 4 → **Go to question 9**

About once a month ☐ 5

Only a few times a year ☐ 6

I never drink alcohol now ☐ 7

Q9   When did you **last** have an alcoholic drink or alcopop?

Tick one box
1080

Today   ☐ 1 ┐
Yesterday   ☐ 2 ├→ **Go to question 10**
Some other time during the last week   ☐ 3 ┘

1 week, but less than 2 weeks ago   ☐ 4 ┐
2 weeks, but less than 4 weeks ago   ☐ 5 │
1 month, but less than 6 months ago   ☐ 6 ├→ **END**
6 months ago or more   ☐ 7 ┘

Q10 Which, if any, of the drinks shown below, have you drunk in the last 7 days?
Please (✓) either yes or no for each kind of drink.
For each kind of drink, write in the box how much you drank in the <u>last 7 days</u>.

**Beer, lager cider or shandy
(exclude bottles or cans of shandy)**

Have you drunk this in <u>the last 7 days</u>?

Tick one box
1081

No   ☐ 2 → **Go to question 11**

Yes   ☐ 1 ┐
              ↓

How much did you drink in the <u>last 7 days</u>?
Write in:

Spare 1082

1083 - 1086
☐   **Pints** (if half a pint, write in ½)

Spare 1087

1088 - 1089
AND/OR ☐   **Large cans or bottles**

Spare 1090

1091 - 1092
AND/OR ☐   **Small cans or bottles**

Q11 **Spirits or liqueurs, such as gin, vodka, whisky, rum, brandy or cocktails**

Have you drunk this in <u>the last 7 days</u>?

Tick one box

1093

No [2] → **Go to question 12**

Yes [1]

How much did you drink in the <u>last 7 days?</u>
Write in:

Spare 1094

1095 - 1096

[ ] **Glasses (count doubles as two glasses)**

Q12 **Sherry or martini (including port, vermouth, cinzano, dubonnet)**

Have you drunk this in <u>the last 7 days</u>?

Tick one box

1097

No [2] → **Go to question 13**

Yes [1]

How much did you drink in the <u>last 7 days?</u>
Write in:

Spare 1098

1099 - 1100

[ ] **Glasses (count doubles as two glasses)**

Q13 **Wine (including babycham and champagne)**

Have you drunk this in <u>the last 7 days</u>?

Tick one box

1101

No [2] → **Go to question 14**

Yes [1]

How much did you drink in the <u>last 7 days?</u>
Write in:

Spare 1102

1103 - 1104

[ ] **Glasses**

Spare 1105-1115

Q14   **Alcopop (such as Bacardi Breezer, Smirnoff Ice, WKD, Reef etc.)**

Have you drunk this in <u>the last 7 days</u>?

Tick one box

1116

No   ☐ 2   → **Go to question 15**

Yes   ☐ 1

How much did you drink in the <u>last 7 days?</u>
Write in:

Spare 1117

1118 - 1119

☐   **Large cans or bottles**

Spare 1120

1121- 1122

AND/OR ☐   **Small cans or bottles**

Q15   **Other kinds of <u>alcoholic</u> drink?**

Have you drunk this in <u>the last 7 days</u>?

Tick one box

1123

No   ☐ 2   → **END**

Yes   ☐ 1   → **Complete details below**

Write in name of drink

How much did you drink in the <u>last 7 days?</u>
Write in:

1124		1125 - 1134
☐	→	☐
1135		1136 - 1145
☐	→	☐
1146		1147 -1156
☐	→	☐

Spare 1157 - 1170

Thank you for answering these questions.

Please give the booklet back to the interviewer.

National Diet and Nutrition Survey

Booklet for Young Adults (16-24 years)

In Confidence

Point	Address	CKL	Person no	First name:	
					1012 - 1026
1001 - 1005	1006 - 1007	1008	1011		

Card	Type	Batch	Interviewer no.	Spare
0 1	3		1032 - 1037	
1009 - 1010	1038	1027 - 1031		1039 - 1050

Example Questions: How to fill in this questionnaire

Most of the questions on the following pages can be answered simply by ticking the box below or alongside the answer that applies to you.

Tick **one** box

Very healthy life	Fairly healthy life	Not very healthy life	An unhealthy life
☐ 1	✓ 2	☐ 3	☐ 4

Example 1: Do you feel that you lead a ...

Sometimes you are asked to write in a number or the answer in your own words. Please enter numbers as figures rather than words.

Example 2:   Write in no.   **6**

On most pages you should answer ALL the questions but sometimes you will find the box you have ticked has an arrow next to it with an instruction to go to another question.

Tick **one** box

Example 3: Would you like to lead a healthier life than you do now?

Yes ✓ 1   **Go to question 4**

No ☐ 2   **Go to question 5**

By following the instructions carefully you will miss out questions which do not apply to you.

PEACH

SMOKING

Q1 Have you ever smoked a cigarette, a cigar or a pipe, or anything with tobacco in it?

Tick one box

1051

Yes ☐ 1 → **Go to question 2**

No ☐ 2 → **Go to question 11 on page 3**

Q2 Have you ever smoked a cigarette?

Tick one box

1052

Yes ☐ 1 → **Go to question 3**

No ☐ 2 → **Go to question 11 on page 3**

Q3 How old were you when you first tried smoking a cigarette, even if it was only a puff or two?

1053 - 1054

Write in how old you were then ☐ → **Go to question 4**

Q4 Do you smoke cigarettes at all nowadays?

Tick one box

1055

Yes ☐ 1 → **Go to question 6**

No ☐ 2 → **Go to question 5**

Q5 Did you smoke cigarettes regularly or occasionally?

Tick one box

1056

Regularly, that is at least one cigarette a day ☐ 1 → **Go to question 9 on page 2**

Occasionally ☐ 2 → **Go to question 11 on page 3**

I never really smoked cigarettes, just tried them once or twice ☐ 3

CURRENT SMOKERS

Q6 About how many cigarettes a day do you usually smoke on <u>weekdays</u>?

1057 - 1059

Write in number smoked a day ☐ → **Go to question 7**

Q7 And about how many cigarettes a day do you usually smoke at <u>weekends</u>?

1060 - 1062

Write in number smoked a day ☐ → **Go to question 8 on page 2**

Q8   Do you <u>mainly</u> smoke ...

Tick one box
1063

filter-tipped cigarettes,   ☐ 1

plain or untipped cigarettes,   ☐ 2   → **Go to question 11**

or hand-rolled cigarettes?   ☐ 3

Q9   About how many cigarettes did you smoke IN A DAY when you smoked them regularly?

1064 - 1066

Write in number smoked a day   ☐   → **Go to question 10**

Q10   How long ago did you stop smoking cigarettes regularly? Was it...

Tick one box
1067

...less than 6 months ago,   ☐ 1

...6 months to 1 year ago,   ☐ 2

...1 to 2 years ago,   ☐ 3   → **Go to question 11**

...2 to 5 years ago,   ☐ 4

...5 to 10 years ago,   ☐ 5

...or more than 10 years ago,   ☐ 6

Spare 1068 - 1074

DRINKING

EVERYONE PLEASE ANSWER

Q11 Do you ever drink alcohol nowadays, including drinks you brew or make at home?

Tick one box

1075

Yes ☐ 1 → **Go to question 14**

No ☐ 2 → **Go to question 12**

Q12 Just to check, does that mean you never have an alcoholic drink nowadays, or do you have an alcoholic drink very occasionally, perhaps for medicinal purposes or on special occasions like Christmas and New Year?

Tick one box

1076

Very occasionally ☐ 1 → **Go to question 14**

Never ☐ 2 → **Go to question 13**

Q13 Have you always been a non-drinker or did you stop drinking for some reason?

Tick one box

1077

Always a non-drinker ☐ 1

Used to drink but stopped ☐ 2 → **END**

Q14 How old were you the first time you ever had a proper alcoholic drink?

1078 - 1079

Write in how old you were then ☐ → **Go to question 15**

Q15 Thinking now about all kinds of drinks, how often have you had an alcoholic drink of any kind during the last 12 months?

Tick one box
1080-1081

Almost every day	01	
Five or six days a week	02	
Three or four days a week	03	
Once or twice a week	04	→ **Go to question 16**
Once or twice a month	05	
Once every couple of months	06	
Once or twice a year	07	
Not at all in the last 12 months	08	→ **END**

Q16 Did you have an alcoholic drink in the seven days ending yesterday?

Tick one box
1082

Yes	1	→ **Go to question 17**
No	2	→ **END**

Q17 On how many days out of the last seven did you have an alcoholic drink?

Tick one box
1083

One	1	
Two	2	
Three	3	
Four	4	→ **Go to question 18**
Five	5	
Six	6	
Seven	7	

Q18 Please think about <u>the day in the last week on which you drank the most.</u> (If you drank the same amount on more than one day, please answer about the most recent of those days.)

From this list, please tick all the types of alcoholic drink which you drank <u>on that day</u>. For the ones you drank, write in how much you drank <u>on that day</u>. EXCLUDE NON-ALCOHOLIC OR LOW-ALCOHOL DRINKS, EXCEPT SHANDY.

WRITE IN HOW MUCH DRUNK ON THAT DAY

TICK <u>ALL</u> DRINKS DRUNK ON THAT DAY		Glasses (count doubles as 2 singles)	Pints	Large cans or bottles	Small cans or bottles	
<u>Normal</u> strength beer, lager, stout, cider or shandy (less than 6% alcohol)-exclude bottles/cans of shandy.	1084-1099 ☐ 01		☐	☐	☐	1100-1107
<u>Strong</u> beer, lager, stout or cider (6% alcohol or more, such as Tennants Super, Special Brew, Diamond White)	☐ 02		☐	☐	☐	1108-1115
Spirits or liqueurs, such as gin, whisky, rum, brandy, vodka, or cocktails	☐ 03	☐				1116-1117
Sherry or martini (including port, vermouth, cinzano, dubonnet)	☐ 04	☐				1118-1119

		Large glasses (250ml)	Standard glasses (175ml)	Small glasses (125ml)	Bottles (750ml)	
Wine (including babycham and champagne). You can write in parts of a bottle e.g. half a bottle	☐ 05	☐	☐	☐	☐	1120-1128

					Small cans or bottles	
Alcoholic soft drink ('alcopop') such as Hooch, or a pre-mixed alcoholic drink such as Bacardi Breezer, WKD or Smirnoff Ice	☐ 06				☐	1129-1130

Other kinds of alcoholic drink **WRITE IN NAME OF DRINK**		Glasses (count doubles as 2 singles)	Pints	Large cans or bottles	Small cans or bottles	
1. [_____]	☐ 07	☐	☐	☐	☐	1131-1140
2. [_____]	☐ 08	☐	☐	☐	☐	1141-1150

Spare 1151 - 1170

Thank you for answering these questions.

Please give the booklet back to the interviewer.

Appendix G   Nurse (stage 2) overview and documents

G1   Overview of information collected during the nurse stage

Table G.1 summarises the information collected during the nurse stage. Some of the information collected by nurses was limited to particular age groups.

Table G.1: Information collected during the nurse stage	
Measurement or procedure	**Participant**
Details of prescribed medications	All ages
Blood pressure	Aged 4 years and over
Infant length measurements	Aged 18-23 months
Waist and hip circumferences	Aged 11 years and over
Demi-span[i]	Aged 65 years and over and those aged 16-64 years where height could not be measured
Mid Upper Arm Circumference (MUAC)	Aged 2-15 years
24-hour urine collection	Aged 4 years and over fully out of nappies
Non-fasting blood sampling	Aged 1.5-3 years and diabetics not willing to fast
Fasting blood sampling	Aged 4 years and over

The CAPI nurse interview and documents used during the nurse stage are shown in the remainder of this Appendix.

---

[i] Demi-span was measured in participants for whom, for postural reasons, a measure of height would give a poor measure of stature (e.g. in some elderly people, or for people with certain disabilities). Demi-span is strongly related to a person's height and is the distance between the sternal notch and the finger roots with the arm out-stretched laterally.

National Diet and Nutrition Survey (NDNS)

P8752 Year 3

Program Documentation

Nurse Schedule

This 'paper version of the program' has been created to indicate the wording and content of the interviewer questionnaire.

- Instructions for the nurse are given in capital letters, and questions the interviewer is to ask the respondent are given as normal text.
- Items which appear in the actual program but which have been excluded here for clarity include: Repetition of respondent's name on each question; Checks on the accuracy of answer codes in relation to each other; Prompts for back-coding during the edit process.

Contents:

HOUSEHOLD GRID

Intro
NURSE: The following information is to be taken from page 2 of the NRF.
1 Continue

Name
NURSE: Enter the name of RESPONDENT NUMBER from the NRF.
: STRING [20]

Sex
NURSE: Code the sex of RESPONDENT NUMBER from the NRF.
1 Male
2 Female

AgeOf
NURSE: Enter the age of RESPONDENT NUMBER from the NRF.
: 0..120

AgeOfM
Age in months
: 00..1440

DOB
82709 CAPI_NURSE_v1.1
NURSE: Enter the date of birth of RESPONDENT NUMBER from the NRF.

OC
NURSE: Enter the code for RESPONDENT NUMBER from NRF.
1 Agreed nurse
2 Refused nurse
3 No diary data

DemiS
NURSE: From NRF please say whether RESPONDENT NUMBER requires a demi-span measurement.
1 Yes
2 No

ParName1
NURSE: Enter the name of the 1st parent giving consent for RESPONDENT NUMBER from NRF.
: STRING [20]

ParName2
NURSE: Enter the name of the 2nd parent giving consent for RESPONDENT NUMBER from NRF.
If only 1 parent just press <Enter>
: STRING [20]

BMI
NURSE: From NRF please enter BMI calculation for RESPONDENT NUMBER.
If no BMI available code 'Don't Know' <Ctrl K>
: 5.0..50.0

NURSE SCHEDULE

RName
Name of respondent.
: STRING [20

RAge
Age of respondent.
Range: 0..120

RDoB
DoB of respondent
: DATETYPE

MonthAge
Age of infant respondent (in months).
: 0..97

RDemiS
Requires demi-span?
1   Yes
2   No

WeekAge
Age of infant respondent (in weeks).
: 0..997

RSex
Sex of respondent.
1   Male
2   Female

DrugClot
Any anti-coagulant drugs recorded in the drugs section?
1   Yes
2   No

NSeqNo
Nurse Schedule number.
: 0..2

RefInfo
Name is recorded as having refused a nurse visit.
Please check if he/she has changed his/her mind.
1   Change   "Yes, now agrees to nurse visit"
2   Still   "No, still refuses nurse visit"

Info

NURSE: You are in the Nurse Schedule for...

Person	*(Person number)*
Name	*(Respondent name)*
Age	*(Respondent age* at date of 1st Interviewer visit*)*
DOB	*(Respondent date of birth)*
Sex	*(Respondent sex)*
Height	*(Respondent Height cm)*
Weight	*(Respondent Weight kg)*
BMI	*(Respondent BMI)*

LInfo

1   Yes   "Yes, I will do the interview now"
2   No   "No, I will not be able to do this interview"

InfoS

Safety copy of Info
1   Yes   "Yes, I will do the interview now",
2   No   "No, I will not be able to do this interview"

StrtNur

Start time of the interview
: TIMETYPE

MachDate

Automatically recorded date of interview
: DATETYPE

NEndDate

Date at end of interview
: DATETYPE

DateOK

NURSE : Today's date according to the laptop is *(Date)*.
Is this the correct date?
1   Yes
2   No

NurDate

NURSE: Enter the date of this interview
: DATETYPE

NDoBD

Can I just check your date of birth?
NURSE : Enter day, month and year of (respondent's name)'s date of birth separately.
Enter the **day** here.
: 1..31

NDoBM
NURSE : Enter the code for the **month** of (respondent's name)'s date of birth.
1   January
2   February
3   March
4   April
5   May
6   June
7   July
8   August
9   September
10   October
11   November
12   December

NDoBY
NURSE: Enter the **year** of (respondent's name)'s date of birth.
: 1890..2008

NDoB
Date of birth (derived)
: DATETYPE

DoBDisc
NURSE: Please explain the difference between date of birth the Interviewer recorded (Date of birth of respondent) and date of birth you have just recorded (Date of birth derived).
:OPEN

HHAge
Age of respondent based on Nurse entered date of birth and date at time of household interview.
: 0..120

ConfAge
: 0..120

IF (Age ≤ 15) THEN
CParInt
NURSE: A child can **only** be interviewed with the permission of, and in the presence of, their parent or a person who has (permanent) legal parental responsibility *(specify names)*. No measurements should be carried out without the agreement of both the parent **and** the child.
N.B Written child assent, where appropriate, should also be sought from children who are able to give it.
1   Continue

IF (Age IN 16..49) AND (Sex = Female) THEN
PregNTJ
Can I check, are you pregnant or breastfeeding at the moment?
1   Yes
2   No

HlthCh
(Can I just check,) have there been any changes to you/your child's general health since you/he/she were/was visited by the interviewer?
1   Yes
2   No

If (HlthCh = Yes) THEN
HlthChWh
INTERVIEWER: PLEASE RECORD DETAILS OF THE RESPONDENT'S CHANGE IN GENERAL HEALTH.
: OPEN

IF (PregNTJ = No) THEN
MedCNJD
Are /(Is) you/(child's name) taking or using any medicines, pills, syrups, ointments, puffers or injections prescribed for you (him/her) by a doctor or a nurse?
NURSE: If statins have been prescribed by a doctor please code them here. If they have been bought without a prescription code at Statins question
NURSE: INCLUDE DIETARY SUPPLEMENTS AS LONG AS PRESCRIBED.
MEDICINES SHOULD BE BEING TAKEN NOW, OR BE CURRENT PRESCRIPTIONS FOR USE 'AS REQUIRED.'
1   Yes
2   No

IF (Age >= 16) AND (MedCNJD = No) THEN
Statins
Are you taking statins (drugs to lower cholesterol) bought over the counter from a pharmacist, without the prescription of a doctor?
1   Yes
2   No

IF (Statins = Yes) THEN
StatinA
Have you taken/used any statins in the last 7 days?
1   Yes
2   No

IF (MedCNJD = Yes) THEN
MedIntro
Could I take down the names of the medicines, including pills, syrups, ointments, puffers or injections, prescribed for you/(child's name) by a doctor?
1   Continue

DrCod1
NURSE: To do the drug coding now, press <Ctrl Enter>, select *(DrugCode)* with the highlight bar and press <Enter>.
1   Continue

IF (Sex = Female) AND (Age = 10-15) THEN
UPreg
NURSE: Has the respondent (or her parent) told you that she is pregnant or breastfeeding?
Do **not** ask for this information - only code whether or not it has been volunteered.
1   Pregnant   "Yes, told me she is pregnant/breastfeeding"
2   NotTold   "No, **not** told me she is pregnant/breastfeeding"

NoBP
NURSE: No blood pressure reading to be done.
Press <1> and <Enter> to continue.
1   Continue

IF (PregNTJ = Yes) OR (UPreg = Pregnant) THEN
PregMes
NURSE: Respondent is pregnant.
No measurements to be done.
1   Continue

NoCodes
NURSE: No blood to be taken.
- Circle consent codes 12, 14, 16, 18 on front of the Consent Booklet.
Press <1> and <Enter> to continue.
1   Continue

(Age = 0-4) OR (IF PregNTJ = Yes) OR (IF UPreg = Pregnant)
IF no NoCodeB = RESPONSE, THEN WE SHOULD ROUTE NURSES TO "THANKS"
and route them out of the CAPI
NoCodeB
NURSE: NO MEASUREMENTS TO BE TAKEN.
-Circle codes 02, 04, 06, 08, 10, 12, 14, 16, 18, on the front of the Consent Booklet.
Press <1> and <Enter> to continue."
1   Continue

AllCheck
Check before leaving the respondent:
That *(respondent's name)* has a Consent Booklet.
That full GP details are entered on front of the Office Consent Booklet.
The name by which GP knows respondent.
That all details are completed on front of the Office Consent Booklet.
That all necessary signatures have been collected in both consent booklets.
That appropriate codes have been ringed on the front of the office consent booklet.
(For those who have agreed a return visit to either give a blood samples or a 24 urine sample, there will be further consents to collect at the return visit).
Press <1> and <Enter> to continue.
1   Continue

EndReach
NURSE: End of questionnaire reached
Press <1> and <Enter> to continue."
1   Continue

NurOut
NURSE: Why were you not able to complete the nurse schedule for person *(Person Number: Respondent Name)*?

Thank
NURSE: Thank respondent for his/her co-operation.
Then press <1> and <Enter> to finish.
1   Continue

INFANT LENGTH
FOR RESPONDENTS AGED 18 MONTHS TO 2 YEARS

IF (Age < 2) THEN
LgthMod
NURSE: Now follows the **Infant Length** module.
1   Continue

LgthInt
(As I mentioned earlier,) I would like to measure *(child's name)'s* length.
IF ASKED: This gives us information about your child's growth.
1   Agree   "Length measurement agreed"
2   Refuse   "Length measurement refused"
3   Unable   "Unable to measure length for other reason"

IF (LgthInt = Agree) THEN
Length
NURSE: Measure infant's length and record in centimetres.
If measurement not obtained, enter '999.9'.
Range: 40.0..999.9

IF (Length <> 999.9) THEN
LgthRel
NURSE: Is this measurement reliable?
1   Yes
2   No

IF (Length=999.9) THEN
YNoLgth
NURSE: Give reason for not obtaining a length measurement
1   Refuse   "Measurement refused"
2   TryNot   "Attempted, not obtained"
3   NoTry   "Measurement not attempted"

IF (YNoLgth = Refuse.. TryNot or NoTry) OR (LgthInt = Refuse OR Unable) THEN
NoAttL
NURSE: Give reason for *(refusal/not obtaining measurement/not attempting the measurement)*.
1   Asleep   "Child asleep"
2   Fright   "Child too frightened or upset"
3   Shy   "Child too shy"
4   Lie   "Child would not lie still"
95   Other   "Other reason(s)"

IF (NoAttL = Other) THEN
OthNLth
NURSE: Enter details of other reason(s) for not obtaining/attempting the length measurement.
: STRING [100]

IF (Length <> 999.9) THEN
MbkLgth
NURSE: Write the results of the length measurement on respondent's Measurement Record Card.
1   Continue

PRESCRIBED MEDICATIONS

{Following questions asked as a loop:}

IF (MedCNJD = Yes) THEN
MedBI
NURSE: Enter name of drug no
Ask if you can see the containers for all prescribed medicines currently being taken.
If Aspirin, record dosage as well as name."
: STRING[50]

MedBIA
Have/(Has) you/(child's name) taken/used *(text from MedBI)* in the last 7 days?
1   Yes
2   No

MedBIC
NURSE CHECK: Any more drugs to enter?
1   Yes
2   No

MID-UPPER ARM CIRCUMFERENCE
FOR RESPONDENTS AGED 15 AND UNDER

IF (Age <15) AND (UPreg = NO) THEN
MUACInt
(As I mentioned earlier,) I would like to measure your/(respondent's name)'s upper arm circumference.
NURSE: **IF ASKED:** This gives us information about the distribution of fat.
1   Agree   "Respondent agrees to have upper arm circumference measured"
2   Refuse   "Respondent refuses to have upper arm circumference measured"
3   Unable   "Unable to measure upper arm circumference for reason other
     than refusal"

IF (MUACInt = Agree) THEN
CUpArm
NURSE: Measure circumference of non-dominant arm and record in centimetres.
If measurement not obtained, enter '99.9'
: 5.0..100.0

IF (CUpArm = 5.0..99.8) THEN
CUpRel
Is the *(first/second/third)* measurement reliable?
1   Yes
2   No

IF (CUpArm = 99.9 *(both attempts)*) THEN
CRespUp
NURSE CHECK:
1   Refused   "Both measurements refused"
2   TryNot   "Attempted not obtained"
3   NoTry   "Measurement not attempted"

IF (CUpArm <> 99.9 *(both attempts)*) THEN
CUpMeas
NURSE CHECK: Arm circumference measured with respondent:
1   Standing   "Standing"
2   Sitting   "Sitting"
3   Lying   "Lying down"

CWhArm
NURSE: Did you take the measurement from the dominant or non-dominant arm?
1   Dominant,
2   Non-dominant (if not measured from right arm enter in memo/remark)

IF (CRespUp = Refused OR TryNot OR NoTry) OR (CUpArm = 99.9) THEN
NoCUpArm
NURSE: Give reason(s) for *(only obtaining one measurement/refusal/not obtaining measurement/measurement not being attempted.*"
: STRING [140]

IF (CUpArm = 5.0..99.8) THEN
ArmRes
NURSE: Offer to write results of arm circumference measurement on respondent's
Measurement Record Card. Complete new card if required.
1   Continue

BLOOD PRESSURE
FOR RESPONDENTS AGED 5 AND OVER WHO ARE NOT PREGNANT

ASK ALL AGED 5+ EXCEPT PREGNANT WOMEN
BPMod
NURSE: Now follows the **Blood Pressure** module.
1   Continue

IF (Age >15) THEN
BPIntro
(As I mentioned earlier) We would like to measure your/(child's name)'s blood pressure.
The analysis of blood pressure readings will tell us a lot about the health of the
population.
1   Continue

IF (Age 5 -15) THEN
BPBlurb
NURSE:··Read out to parent *(if applicable)*:
(As I mentioned earlier) we would like to measure your/(child's name)'s blood pressure.
If you wish, I will write the results on your/(his/her) Measurement Record Card.
I will not, however, be able to tell you what the results mean. This has to be calculated
using your/(his/her) age, sex and height. Also blood pressure can vary from day to day
and throughout the day, so one high reading would not necessarily mean that
you/(he/she) have/(has) high blood pressure.
However, if you would like us to, we will send your/(his/her) results to your/(his/her) GP
who is better placed to interpret them.
In the unlikely event that (respondent's name) should be found to have a high blood
pressure for your/(his/her) age and height, we shall advise your/(his/her) GP (with your
permission) that your/(his/her) blood pressure should be measured again.
1   Continue

BPConst
NURSE: Does the respondent agree to blood pressure measurement?
1   Agree   "Yes, agrees"
2   Refuse   "No, refuses"
3   Unable   "Unable to measure BP for reason other than refusal"

IF (BPConst = Agree) AND (Age >=13) THEN
ConSubX
May I just check, have you eaten, smoked, drunk alcohol or done any (vigorous)
exercise in the past 30 minutes?
CODE ALL THAT APPLY.
1   Eat   "Eaten"
2   Smoke   "Smoked"
3   Drink   "Drunk alcohol"
4   Exercise   "Done (vigorous) exercise"
5   None   "(None of these)"

IF (BPConst = Agree) AND (Age 5 - 12) THEN
ConSubX2
May I just check, has (respondent's name) eaten, or done any vigorous exercise, in the past 30 minutes?
CODE ALL THAT APPLY.
1   Eat   "Eaten"
2   Exercise   "Done vigorous exercise"
3   None   "Neither"

DINNo
NURSE: Please record the Omron serial number.
: 001..999

CufSize
NURSE: Select cuff and attach to the respondent's **right** arm.
Ask the respondent to sit still for five minutes.
READ OUT: 'I am going to leave you to sit quietly now for 5 minutes. During that time you must not read and your legs are to remain uncrossed. After the 5 minutes, I will carry out 3 recordings with a minute between them. While I am doing these recordings I will not speak to you, and you must not speak to me. Once I have completed the recordings I will tell you what they are.'
Record cuff size chosen.
1   Small   "Small (15-22 cm)"
2   Medium   "Medium (22-32 cm)"
3   Large   "Large (32-42 cm)"

Sys to Pulse repeated for up to three blood pressure readings

Sys
NURSE: Enter the *(first/second/third)* **systolic reading** (mmHg).
If reading not obtained, enter 999.
: 001..999

Dias
NURSE: Enter the *(first/second/third)* **diastolic reading** (mmHg).
If reading not obtained, enter 999.
: 001..999

Pulse
NURSE: Enter the *(first/second/third)* **pulse reading** (bpm).
If reading not obtained, enter 999.
: 001..999

Full
All readings OK
1   Yes
2   No

IF (AT LEAST ONE '999' RESPONSE) THEN
YNoBP
NURSE: Enter reason for not recording any full BP readings.

1	Tried	"Blood pressure measurement attempted but not obtained"
2	NoTry	"Blood pressure measurement not attempted"
3	Refused	"Blood pressure measurement refused"

RespBPS

1	Three	"Three"
2	Two	"Two"
3	One	"One"
4	Tried	"Tried"
5	NoTry	"NoTry"
6	Refused	"Refused"

IF (RespBPS = Two..Refused) OR (BPConst = Refuse) THEN
NAttBPD
NURSE: Record why *(only two readings obtained/only one reading obtained/reading not obtained/reading not attempted/reading refused/unable to take reading)*.
CODE ALL THAT APPLY.

1	PC	"Problems with PC"
2	Upset	"Respondent upset/anxious/nervous"
3	Error844	"Error 844' reading"
4	Shy	"Too shy *(children)*"
5	Fidget	"Child would not sit still long enough *(children)*"
6	Other	"Other reason(s) (specify at next question)"
7	Cuff	"Problems with Cuff fitting/painful"
8	Omron	"Problems with Omron readings (zeros, no readings)"
9	Laptop	"Problems with laptop"

IF (NAttBPD = Other) THEN
OthNBP
NURSE: Enter full details of other reason(s) for not obtaining/attempting three BP readings.
: STRING [140]

IF (RespBPS = One, Two or Three) THEN
DifBPC
NURSE: Record any problems taking readings.
CODE ALL THAT APPLY.

1	NoProb	"No problems taking blood pressure"
2	LeftOnly	"Reading taken on left arm because right arm not suitable"
3	Upset	"Respondent was upset/anxious/nervous"
4	Other	"Other problems (specify at next question)"
5	Cuff	"Problems with cuff fitting/painful"
6	Omron	"Problems with Omron readings (zeros, no readings)"

IF (DifBPC = Other) THEN
OthDifBP
NURSE: Record full details of other problem(s) taking readings.
: STRING [140]

IF (RespBPS = One, Two or Three) THEN
GPRegBP
Are/(Is) you/(child's name) registered with a GP?
1   Yes
2   No
IF (GPRegBP = Yes) THEN
GPSend
May we send your/(child's name)'s blood pressure readings to your/(his/her) GP?
1   Yes
2   No

IF (GPSend = No) THEN
GPRefC
NURSE: Specify reason(s) for refusal to allow BP readings to be sent to GP.
CODE ALL THAT APPLY.
1   NeverSee   "Hardly/Never sees GP"
2   GPKnows   "GP knows respondent's BP level"
3   Bother   "Does not want to bother GP"
4   Other   "Other (specify at next question)"

IF (GPRefC = Other) THEN
OthRefC
NURSE: Give full details of reason(s) for refusal.
: STRING [140]

IF (GPReg <> Yes) OR (GPSend = No) THEN
Code02
NURSE: Circle consent **code 02** on front of Consent Booklet.
1   Continue

IF (GPSend = Yes) THEN
Code01
NURSE:
a) Complete 'Blood pressure to GP in both the Consent Booklet and the Respondent Copy.
b) Ask respondent/(respondent's parent) to read, sign and date the form in both the Consent Booklet and the Respondent Copy.
c) Check that GP name, address and phone no. are recorded on the Consent Form.
d) Check the name by which GP knows respondent.
e) Circle consent **code 01** on front of the Consent Booklet.
1   Continue

IF (RespBPS = One, Two or Three) THEN
BPOffer
NURSE: Offer blood pressure results to respondent/(respondent's parent).
(Displays readings)

Enter these on (respondent's name)'s **Measurement Record Card** (complete new record card if required).
1   Continue

DEMI-SPAN
FOR ALL RESPONDENTS AGED 65 AND OVER OR THOSE WITH AN UNRELIABLE HEIGHT MEASUREMENT

ASK ALL AGED 65+ OR AGED 16-64 WITH UNRELIABLE HEIGHT MEASUREMENT
SpanIntro
NURSE: Now follows the **Measurement of Demi-span**.
1   Continue

SpanInt
I would now like to measure the length of your arm. Like height, it is an indicator of size.
NURSE CODE:
1	Agree	"Respondent agrees to have demi-span measured"
2	Refuse	"Respondent refuses to have demi-span measured"
3	Unable	"Unable to measure demi-span for reason other than refusal"

Repeat for up to three demi-span measurements.
Third measurement taken only if first two measurements differ by more than 3cm.

IF (SpanInt = Agree) THEN
Span
NURSE: Enter the *(first/second/third)* demi-span measurement in centimetres.
If measurement not obtained, enter '999.9'.
Range: 5.0..1000.0

IF (Span <> 999.9) THEN
SpanRel
NURSE: Is the *(first/second/third)* measurement reliable?
1   Yes
2   No

IF (Span = 999.9 *(both attempts)*) THEN
YNoSpan
NURSE: Give reason for not obtaining at least one demi-span measurement.
1	Refuse	"Measurement refused"
2	TryNot	"Attempted but not obtained"
3	NoTry	"Measurement not attempted"

IF (YNoSpan = Refuse OR TryNot OR NoTry) THEN
NotAttM
NURSE: Give reason for *(refusal/not obtaining measurement/measurement not being attempted)*.
1	Bent	"Cannot straighten arms"
2	Bed	"Respondent confined to bed"
3	Stoop	"Respondent too stooped"
4	NotUnd	"Respondent did not understand the procedure"
5	Other	"Other"

IF (NotAttM = Other) THEN
OthAttM
NURSE: Give full details of other reason for *(refusal/not obtaining measurement/measurement not being attempted)*.
: STRING [140]

IF (Span <> 999.9) THEN
SpnM
NURSE CHECK: Demi-span was measured with the respondent:
CODE ALL THAT APPLY.
1	Wall	"Standing against the wall"
2	NoWall	"Standing not against the wall"
3	Sitting	
4	Lying	"Lying down"
5	LeftArm	"Demi-span measured on left arm due to unsuitable right arm"

IF (Span <> 999.9) THEN
DSCard
NURSE: Write results of demi-span measurement on respondent's Measurement Record Card.
1   Continue

WAIST AND HIP
FOR RESPONDENTS AGED 11 AND OVER WHO ARE NOT PREGNANT

ASK ALL RESPONDENTS AGED 11+ EXCEPT PREGNANT WOMEN
WHMod
NURSE: Now follows the **Waist and Hip Circumference Measurement**.
1   Continue

WHIntro
I would now like to measure your waist and hips. The waist relative to hip measurement
is very useful for assessing the distribution of weight over the body.
NURSE CODE:
1   Agree   "Respondent agrees to have waist/hip ratio measured"
2   Refuse   "Respondent refuses to have waist/hip ratio measured"
3   Unable   "Unable to measure waist/hip ratio for reason other than refusal"

Repeat for up to three waist-hip measurements.
Third measurement taken only if first two measurements differ by more than 3cm.

IF (WHIntro = Agree) THEN
Waist
NURSE: Measure the waist and hip circumferences **to the nearest mm**.
Enter the *(first/second/third)* waist measurement in centimetres.
(Remember to include the decimal point.)
If measurement not obtained, enter '999.9'.
Range: 40.0..1000.0

IF (WHIntro = Agree) THEN
Hip
NURSE: Measure the waist and hip circumferences **to the nearest mm**.
Enter the *(first/second/third)* measurement of hip circumference in centimetres.
(Remember to include the decimal point.)
If measurement not obtained, enter '999.9'.
Range: 50.0..1000.0

IF (WHIntro = Agree) THEN
RespWH
Imputed
1   Both   "Both obtained"
2   One   "One obtained"
3   Refused   "Refused"
4   NoTry   "NoTry"

IF (Waist = 999.9 *(either attempt)*) OR (Hip = 999.9 *(either attempt)*) THEN
YNoWH
NURSE: Enter reason for not getting both measurements.
1   Refused   "Both measurements refused"
2   TryNot   "Attempted but not obtained"
3   NoTry   "Measurement not attempted"

IF (RespWH = One OR Refused OR NoTry) OR (YNoWH = Refused) THEN
WHPNABM
NURSE: Give reason(s) *(for refusal/why unable/for not obtaining measurement/for not attempting/why only one measurement obtained).*
CODE ALL THAT APPLY.

1	ChairBnd	"Respondent is chairbound"
2	Bed	"Respondent is confined to bed"
3	Stoop	"Respondent is too stooped"
4	NotUnd	"Respondent did not understand the procedure"
5	Other	"Other (SPECIFY AT NEXT QUESTION)"

IF (WHPNABM = OthWH) THEN
OthWH
NURSE: Give full details of 'other' reason(s) for not getting full waist/hip measurement.
: STRING [140]

IF AT LEAST ONE WAIST MEASUREMENT OBTAINED (IF (Waist (1st) <> 999.9 AND Waist (1st) <> EMPTY) OR (Waist (2nd) <> 999.9 AND Waist (2nd) <> EMPTY)) THEN
WJRel
NURSE: Record any problems with **waist** measurement:

1	NoProb	"No problems experienced, **reliable** waist measurement"
2	ProbRel	"Problems experienced - waist measurement **likely to be reliable**"
3	ProbSlUn	"Problems experienced - waist measurement likely to be **slightly unreliable**"
4	ProbUn	"Problems experienced - waist measurement **likely to be unreliable**"

IF (WJRel = ProbRel OR ProbSlUn OR ProbUn) THEN
ProbWJ
NURSE: Record whether problems experienced are likely to increase or decrease the **waist** measurement.

1	Increase	"Increases measurement"
2	Decrease	"Decreases measurement"

IF AT LEAST ONE HIP MEASUREMENT OBTAINED IF ((Hip (1st) <> 999.9 AND Hip (1st) <> EMPTY) OR (Hip (2nd) <> 999.9 AND Hip (2nd) <> EMPTY)) THEN
HJRel
NURSE: Record any problems with **hip** measurement:

1	NoProb	"No problems experienced, **reliable** hip measurement"
2	ProbRel	"Problems experienced - hip measurement likely to be **reliable**"
3	ProbSlUn	"Problems experienced - hip measurement likely to be **slightly unreliable**"
4	ProbUn	"Problems experienced - hip measurement likely to be **unreliable**"

IF (HJRel = ProbRel OR ProbSlUn OR ProbUn) THEN
ProbHJ
NURSE: Record whether problems experienced are likely to increase or decrease the hip measurement.

1	Increase	"Increases measurement"
2	Decrease	"Decreases measurement"

IF (RespWH = Both OR One) THEN
WHRes
NURSE: Offer to write results of waist and hip measurements, where applicable, onto respondent's Measurement Record Card.
1   Continue

BMI TO GP CONSENT

IF (GPRegBP <> Yes) THEN
GPRegBM
NURSE CHECK: Is respondent registered with a GP?
1	Yes	"Respondent registered with GP"
2	No	"Respondent not registered with GP"

ConsBMI
During the first stage, the interviewer measured your height and weight and from this, your Body Mass Index (BMI) was calculated. BMI is a way of telling if you're a healthy weight for your height.
May we send your BMI calculation to your GP?
1   Yes
2   No

IF (ConsBMI = Yes) THEN
Code03
NURSE: Obtain signature in both the Consent Booklet and the Respondent Copy.
Circle consent **code 03** on front of the Consent Booklet.
1   Continue

IF (ConsBMI = No) THEN
Code04
"NURSE: The respondent does **not** want their BMI calculation sent to their GP.
Circle consent **code 04** on front of the Consent Booklet.
1   Continue

URINE INTRODUCTION
FOR ALL RESPONDENTS AGED 4 AND OVER (AND NOT IN NAPPIES) WHO ARE NOT PREGNANT

UrDisp
NURSE: NOW FOLLOWS THE 24 HOUR URINE MODULE.
1   Continue

IF (PAge >=13) THEN
UrInt
We are interested in measuring useful diet indicators in the urine such as sodium, potassium, urea and nitrogen. To do this we would like to collect a sample of your urine over a 24 hour period. We cannot get this information from your food diary or in any other way.
1   Continue

If (PAge = 4-12) THEN
UrIntC
We are interested in measuring useful diet indicators in the urine such as sodium, potassium, urea and nitrogen. To do this we would like to collect a sample of (child's name) urine over a 24 hour period. We cannot get this information from their food diary or in any other way.
1   Continue

IF (PAge = 4- 6) THEN
Nappies
Does (child's name) wear nappies at all nowadays?
NURSE: EVEN IF CHILD JUST WEARS NAPPIES AT NIGHT, CODE AS 'Yes'.
1   Yes
2   No

IF (PAge > 6) OR (PAge = 4-6 AND Nappies = No) THEN
UrLeaf1
To make sure that we can measure diet indicators accurately, we need to collect all urine passed within a 24 hour period. Please read this leaflet, it explains about what it involves.
NURSE: EXPLAIN ABOUT THE MEASUREMENT AND GIVE LEAFLET TO RESPONDENT. ALLOW THEM TIME TO READ IT AND ASK ANY QUESTIONS.
1   Continue

IF (PAge >=13) THEN
UrCons
Are you willing to participate in the 24 hour urine sample?
1   Yes
2   No

IF (PAge = 4-12) THEN
UrPCons
And are you willing for (child's name) to participate in the 24 hour urine sample?
1   Yes
2   No

IF (UrCons = Yes) OR (UrPCons = Yes) THEN
PABAInt
NURSE: THE NEXT COUPLE OF QUESTIONS ARE TO DETERMINE IF IT IS
SAFE FOR THE RESPONDENT TO TAKE PABA TABLETS.
1   Continue

UrChk1
NURSE: HAS THE RESPONDENT TOLD YOU THAT THEY ARE TAKING ANY OF
THE FOLLOWING?
…Co-Trimoxazole   BNF CODE 50108
…Septrin   BNF CODE 50108
…Sulfadiazine   BNF CODE 50108
…Trimethoprim   BNF CODE 50108
…Sulfamethoxazole   BNF CODE 50108
…Monotrim   BNF CODE 50108
…Sultrin   BNF CODE 70202
(THESE ARE ALL SULHPONAMIDES)
1   Yes
2   No

IF (UrChk1 = No) THEN
UrChk2
Can I check, are/(is) you/(child's name) allergic to any of the following things?
 - hair dye
 - sunscreen
 - vitamins
1   Yes
2   No

IF (UrChk1 = Yes) or (UrChk2 = Yes) THEN
NoPABA1
NURSE: THIS RESPONDENT MUST NOT TAKE PABA TABLETS BECAUSE THEY
HAVE TOLD YOU THEY ARE (TAKING SULPHONAMIDES) / (TOLD YOU THEY
ARE ALLERGIC TO HAIR DYE, SUNSCREEN OR VITAMINS) / (NOT BEEN ABLE
TO TELL YOU IF THEY ARE TAKING SULPHONAMIDES) / (NOT BEEN ABLE TO
TELL YOU IF THEY ARE ALLERGIC TO HAIR DYE, SUNSCREEN OR VITAMINS).
THIS PERSON CAN STILL GIVE A 24 HOUR SAMPLE BUT SHOULD NOT BE
GIVEN PABA. RING CONSENT CODE 06 AT QUESTION 9 ON THE FRONT OF
THE OFFICE CONSENT BOOKLET.
1   Continue

IF (UrChk1 = No) or (UrChk2 = No) THEN
UrPABA
To make sure that we can measure diet indicators accurately, we need to collect all
urine passed within a 24 hour period. This also involves taking three tablets called
PABA within the same period so we can see how complete the urine sample is.
Please read this leaflet, it explains about what it involves.
NURSE: EXPLAIN ABOUT THE PABA TABLETS AND CONTRAINDICATIONS FOR
USE. GIVE PABA INFORMATION LEAFLET TO RESPONDENT. ALLOW THEM
TIME TO READ IT AND ASK ANY QUESTIONS.
1   Continue

IF (PAge >= 16) THEN
UPABCon
NURSE: IS THE RESPONDENT WILLING TO TAKE PABA TABLETS?

1   Yes
2   No

IF (PAge <16) THEN
UPABPCon
NURSE: IS THE PARENT OR LEGAL GUARDIAN WILLING FOR CHILD TO TAKE
PABA TABLETS?
1   Yes
2   No

If (UPABCon = Yes) OR (UPABPCon = Yes)
PABAPck
NURSE: EXPLAIN TO THE RESPONDENT THAT YOU WILL NEED TO COLLECT
THE PABA PACKAGING WHEN YOU COME BACK TO SUB-SAMPLE THEIR
URINE. THIS IS JUST SO THAT YOU CAN SEND IT BACK TO HNR SO THEY
CAN BE SURE HOW MANY TABLETS WERE TAKEN AND CAN THEREFORE
ANALYSE THE URINE ACCURATELY.
1   Continue

IF (UPABCon = Yes) THEN
UPABCon1
NURSE: EXPLAIN THE NEED FOR WRITTEN CONSENT TO TAKE PABA.ASK
RESPONDENT TO INITIAL FIRST BOX IN '24 HOUR URINE CONSENTS'
SECTION IN THE OFFICE CONSENT BOOKLET AND THE PERSONAL CONSENT
BOOKLET. ASK RESPONDENT TO SIGN AND DATE AT THE BOTTOM OF THE
PAGE IN BOTH COPIES (IF NOT ALREADY DONE).
1   Yes   "Written consent obtained for PABA"
2   No   "Written consent not obtained for PABA"

IF (UPABPCon = Yes) THEN
UPABCon2
NURSE: EXPLAIN THE NEED FOR WRITTEN CONSENT TO TAKE PABA.
ASK PARENT/LEGAL GUARDIAN TO INITIAL FIRST BOX IN '24 HOUR URINE
CONSENTS' SECTION IN THE OFFICE CONSENT BOOKLET AND THE
PERSONAL CONSENT BOOKLET.
ASK PARENT/LEGAL GUARDIAN TO SIGN AND DATE AT THE BOTTOM OF THE
PAGE IN BOTH COPIES (IF NOT ALREADY DONE).
1   Yes   "Written consent obtained for PABA"
2   No   "Written consent not obtained for PABA"

IF (UPABCon = No) OR (UPABCon1 = No) OR (UPABCon2 = No) THEN
NoPABA2
NURSE: THIS RESPONDENT HAS NOT CONSENTED TO TAKE PABA.
THIS PERSON CAN STILL GIVE A 24 HOUR SAMPLE BUT SHOULD NOT BE
GIVEN PABA. RING CONSENT CODE 06 ON THE FRONT OF THE OFFICE
CONSENT BOOKLET.
1   Continue

IF (PAge >= 16) AND (UrCons = Yes) THEN
ULABCon1
NURSE: EXPLAIN THE NEED FOR WRITTEN CONSENT FOR LABORATORY
ANALYSIS OF URINE SAMPLE.
ASK RESPONDENT TO INITIAL SECOND BOX IN '24 HOUR URINE. CONSENTS'
SECTION IN THE OFFICE CONSENT BOOKLET AND THE PERSONAL CONSENT
BOOKLET.

ASK RESPONDENT TO SIGN AND DATE AT THE BOTTOM OF THE PAGE IN BOTH COPIES (IF NOT ALREADY DONE).

1	Yes	"Written consent obtained for lab analysis"
2	No	"Written consent not obtained for lab analysis"

IF (UrCons = Yes) OR (UrPCons = Yes) THEN
ULABCon2
NURSE: EXPLAIN THE NEED FOR WRITTEN CONSENT FOR LABORATORY ANALYSIS OF URINE SAMPLE.
ASK PARENT/LEGAL GUARDIAN TO INITIAL SECOND BOX IN '24 HOUR URINE CONSENTS' SECTION IN THE OFFICE CONSENT BOOKLET AND THE PERSONAL CONSENT BOOKLET.
ASK PARENT/LEGAL GUARDIAN TO SIGN AND DATE AT THE BOTTOM OF THE PAGE IN BOTH COPIES (IF NOT ALREADY DONE).

1	Yes	"Written consent obtained for lab analysis"
2	No	"Written consent not obtained for lab analysis"

IF ((PAge >= 16) AND (UPABCon = Yes)) OR ((PAge < 16) AND (UPABPCon = Yes)) THEN
Code05
NURSE: CIRCLE CONSENT CODE 05 (CONSENT TO TAKE PABA) AT QUESTION 9 ON FRONT OF THE OFFICE CONSENT BOOKLET.
1   Continue

IF ((PAge >= 16) AND (UPABCon = No)) OR ((PAge < 16) AND (UPABPCon = No)) THEN
Code06
NURSE: CIRCLE CONSENT CODE 06 (NO CONSENT TO TAKE PABA) AT QUESTION 9 ON FRONT OF THE OFFICE CONSENT BOOKLET.
1   Continue

IF ((PAge >= 16) AND (ULabCon1 = Yes)) OR ((PAge < 16) AND (ULabCon2 = Yes)) THEN
Code07
NURSE: CIRCLE CONSENT CODE 07 (CONSENT FOR LAB ANALYSIS) AT QUESTION 9 ON FRONT OF THE OFFICE CONSENT BOOKLET.
1   Continue

IF ((PAge >= 16) AND (ULabCon1 = No)) OR ((PAge < 16) AND (ULabCon2 = No)) THEN
Code08
NURSE: CIRCLE CONSENT CODE 08 (NO CONSENT FOR LAB ANALYSIS) AT QUESTION 9 ON FRONT OF OFFICE CONSENT BOOKLET.
1   Continue

IF (ULabCon1 = Yes) OR (ULabCon2 = Yes) THEN
UrExpl
NURSE: MAKE SURE YOU HAVE EXPLAINED ALL PROCEDURES AND PROTOCOLS ABOUT WHAT IS INVOLVED FULLY TO THE RESPONDENT OR PARENT/LEGAL GUARDIAN.
1   Continue

UrAppt
NURSE: PLEASE DO THE FOLLOWING....

1) AGREE A DATE WITH THE RESPONDENT WHEN THEY WILL COLLECT
URINE FOR 24 HOURS (STARTING COLLECTION ON ANY DAY EXCEPT A
THURSDAY).
2) MAKE AN APPOINTMENT WITH THE RESPONDENT TO COLLECT THEIR
SAMPLE, IDEALLY ON EITHER THE DAY THEY STOP COLLECTING URINE
OR THE FOLLOWING DAY (i.e. the day after collection finished). SCHOOL AGED
CHILDREN SHOULD ALWAYS BE ASKED TO COLLECT THEIR URINE ON A
NON-SCHOOL DAY.
3) EXPLAIN THE COLLECTION PROTOCOL.
4) IF THE RESPONDENT IS TAKING PABA, REMIND THEM THAT YOU WILL BE
COLLECTING THE PACKAGING AT YOUR RETURN VISIT.
5) COMPLETE SECTION A OF THE 24 HOUR URINE COLLECTION FORM.
6) GIVE THE RESPONDENT THE URINE COLLECTION SHEET AND ASK THEM
TO COMPLETE SECTION B DURING THEIR COLLECTION PERIOD.
1   Continue

IF (Nappies = Yes) OR (UrCons = No) OR (UrPCons = No) OR (ULabCon1 = No)
OR (ULabCon2 = No) THEN
NoUri
NURSE: NO URINE SAMPLE TO BE TAKEN.
CIRCLE CONSENT CODES 06, 08, 10 ON FRONT OF OFFICE CONSENT
BOOKLET.
1   Continue

URINE COLLECTION
FOR ALL RESPONDENTS AGED 4 AND OVER (AND NOT IN NAPPIES) WHO ARE NOT PREGNANT

UrCInt
NURSE: EXPLAIN THAT YOU ARE HERE TO COLLECT THE URINE SAMPLE.
FOLLOW PROTOCOLS TO MIX, WEIGH AND COLLECT 4 ALIQUOTS OF URINE.
1   Continue

UrColl
NURSE: HAS (RESPONDENT'S NAME) PROVIDED A URINE SAMPLE?
1   Yes
2   No

IF (UrColl = Yes) THEN
UrJugs
NURSE: On collection, which containers have urine inside?
1   Five   "5 litre container only"
2   Two   "2 Litre container only"
3   Both   "Both the 5 litre and 2 litre containers"

IF (UrJugs = Five) OR (UrJugs = Both) THEN
UrWt1
NURSE: WEIGH THE 5 LITRE CONTAINER.
Enter the weight of total urine sample. Enter weight in kilograms, with 2 decimal places.
If measurement not obtained, enter '9.99'.
: 0.01..9.99

UrWt2
NURSE: Enter the weight of total urine sample. Enter weight in kilograms, with 2 decimal places. If measurement not obtained, enter '9.99'.
: 0.01..9.99

IF (UrWt1 - UrWt2 > 0.02) THEN
UrWt3
NURSE: Enter the weight of total urine sample. Enter weight in kilograms, with 2 decimal places. If measurement not obtained, enter '9.99'.
0.01..9.99

IF (UrJugs = Two) OR (UrJugs = Both) THEN
Ur2LWt1
NURSE: WEIGH THE 2 LITRE CONTAINER
Enter the weight of total urine sample. Enter weight in kilograms, with 2 decimal places.
If measurement not obtained, enter '9.99'.
0.01..9.99

Ur2LWt2
NURSE: Enter the weight of urine sample from the 2 litre container. Enter weight in kilograms, with 2 decimal places. If measurement not obtained, enter '9.99'.

: 0.01..9.99

IF (Ur2LWt1 - Ur2LWt2 > 0.02) THEN
Ur2LWt3
NURSE: Enter the weight of urine sample from the 2 litre container. Enter weight in kilograms, with 2 decimal places. If measurement not obtained, enter '9.99'.
: 0.01..9.99

UrSDay
On what date did you start your urine collection?
NURSE: Enter day, month and year separately.
Enter the day here.
NURSE: REFER TO THE 24-HOUR URINE COLLECTION SHEET.
: 1..31

UrSMon
Enter the code for the month here.
NURSE: REFER TO THE 24-HOUR URINE COLLECTION SHEET."
1   January
2   February
3   March
4   April
5   May
6   June
7   July
8   August
9   September
10   October
11   November
12   December

UrSYr
Enter the year here.
NURSE: REFER TO THE 24-HOUR URINE COLLECTION SHEET.
: 2008..2019

UrSDate
On what date did you start your urine collection?
: DATETYPE

UrSHrs
At what time did you start your urine collection?
NURSE: Enter hours and minutes separately.
Enter the hours here.
N.B. Please use the 24-hour clock, e.g. for 2pm enter 14, for 12 midnight enter 0.
NURSE: REFER TO THE 24-HOUR URINE COLLECTION SHEET.
: 0..23

UrSMin
Enter the minutes here.
NURSE: REFER TO THE 24-HOUR URINE COLLECTION SHEET.

: 0..59

UrSTime
At what time did you start your urine collection?
: TIMETYPE

UrEDay
On what date did you finish your urine collection?
NURSE: Enter day, month and year separately.
Enter the day here.
NURSE: REFER TO THE 24-HOUR URINE COLLECTION SHEET."
: 1..31

UrEMon
Enter the code for the month here.
NURSE: REFER TO THE 24-HOUR URINE COLLECTION SHEET.
1   January
2   February
3   March
4   April
5   May
6   June
7   July
8   August
9   September
10   October
11   November
12   December

UrEYr
Enter the year here.
NURSE: REFER TO THE 24-HOUR URINE COLLECTION SHEET.
: 2008..2019

UrEDate
On what date did you start your urine collection?
: DATETYPE

UrEHrs
At what time did you finish your urine collection?
NURSE: Enter hours and minutes separately.
Enter the hours here.
N.B. Please use the 24-hour clock, e.g. for 2pm enter 14, for 12 midnight enter 0.
NURSE: REFER TO THE 24-HOUR URINE COLLECTION SHEET.
: 0..23

UrEMin
Enter the minutes here.
NURSE: REFER TO THE 24-HOUR URINE COLLECTION SHEET.
: 0..59

UrETime
At what time did you start your urine collection?
: TIMETYPE

ChkMss
Did you/(child's name) miss collecting any samples during the 24 hour period?
NURSE: REFER TO THE 24-HOUR URINE COLLECTION SHEET.
1   Yes
2   No

IF (ChkMss = Yes) THEN
HowManM
How many did you/(child's name) miss?
NURSE: REFER TO THE 24-HOUR URINE COLLECTION SHEET.
: 1..10

IF (ChkMss = Yes) THEN
DatMssD
Date of *(first/second/third/fourth/fifth)* missed sample.
NURSE: Enter day, month and year separately.
Enter the day here.
NURSE: REFER TO THE 24-HOUR URINE COLLECTION SHEET.
:1..31

DatMssM
Enter the month here.
NURSE: REFER TO THE 24-HOUR URINE COLLECTION SHEET.
1   January
2   February
3   March
4   April
5   May
6   June
7   July
8   August
9   September
10   October
11   November
12   December

DatMssY
Enter the year here.
NURSE: REFER TO THE 24-HOUR URINE COLLECTION SHEET.
: 2008..2019

DatMss
Date of missed sample.
: DATETYPE

TimMssH
Time of *(first/second/third/fourth/fifth)* missed sample.

NURSE: Enter hours and minutes separately.
Enter the hours here.
N.B. Please use the 24-hour clock, e.g. for 2pm enter 14, for 12 midnight enter 0.
NURSE: REFER TO THE 24-HOUR URINE COLLECTION SHEET.
:0..23

TimMssM
Enter the minutes here.
NURSE: REFER TO THE 24-HOUR URINE COLLECTION SHEET.
:0..59

TimMss
Time of missed sample.
:TIMETYPE

IF (UPABCon1 = Yes) OR (UPABCon2 = Yes) THEN
AllPABA
I now need to record information about the PABA tablets you took.
Did you take all three PABA tablets?
NURSE: REFER TO THE 24-HOUR URINE COLLECTION SHEET.
NURSE: PLEASE REMEMBER TO OBTAIN THE PABA BLISTER PACK AND RETURN
IT TO HNR, REGARDLESS OF HOW MANY TABLETS HAVE BEEN TAKEN.
1   Yes
2   No

IF (AllPABA = No) THEN
ChkPABA
Did you/(child's name) take any of the PABA tablets?
NURSE: REFER TO THE 24-HOUR URINE COLLECTION SHEET.
NURSE: PLEASE REMEMBER TO OBTAIN THE PABA BLISTER PACK AND RETURN
IT TO HNR, REGARDLESS OF HOW MANY TABLETS HAVE BEEN TAKEN.
1   Yes
2   No

IF (AllPABA = Yes) OR (ChkPABA = Yes) THEN
DatPABD
Date *(first/second/third)* PABA tablet taken.
NURSE: If *(first/second/third)* PABA tablet not taken enter CTRL/K.
NURSE: Enter day, month and year separately.
Enter the day here.
NURSE: REFER TO THE 24-HOUR URINE COLLECTION SHEET.
:1..31

DatPABM
Enter the month here.
NURSE: REFER TO THE 24-HOUR URINE COLLECTION SHEET.
1   January
2   February
3   March
4   April
5   May

6	June
7	July
8	August
9	September
10	October
11	November
12	December

DatPABY
Enter the year here.
NURSE: REFER TO THE 24-HOUR URINE COLLECTION SHEET.
: 2008..2019

IF (AllPABA = Yes) OR (ChkPABA = Yes) THEN
DatPAB
Date *(first/second/third)* PABA tablet taken
: DATETYPE

TimPABH
Time *(first/second/third)* PABA tablet taken.
NURSE: Enter hours and minutes separately.
Enter the hours here.
N.B. Please use the 24-hour clock, e.g. for 2pm enter 14, for 12 midnight enter 0.
NURSE: REFER TO THE 24-HOUR URINE COLLECTION SHEET.
: 0..23

TimPABM
Enter the minutes here.
NURSE: REFER TO THE 24-HOUR URINE COLLECTION SHEET.
: 0..59

TimPAB
Time PABA tablet taken.
: TIMETYPE

IF (PAge >= 16) THEN
Diet
Were/(was) you/(child's name) taking any dietary supplements on the days you collect the urine sample?
1   Yes
2   No

IF (Diet = Yes) THEN
DWhat
What did you/(child's name) take?
NURSE RECODE NAME OF SUPPLEMENT TAKEN
: STRING[60]

DMore
Any others?
1   Yes

2   No

IF (PAge >= 16) THEN
StrUrA
May we have your consent to store any remaining urine for future analysis?
1   Yes   "Storage consent given"
2   No   "Consent refused"

IF (PAge<16) THEN)
StrUrC
May we have your consent to store any of (child's name)'s remaining urine for future analysis?
1 Yes   "Storage consent given"
2 No   "Consent refused"

IF (StrUrA = Yes) OR (StrUrC = Yes) THEN
Code09
ASK RESPONDENT/(PARENT / LEGAL GUARDIAN) TO INITIAL THIRD BOX IN '24 HOUR URINE CONSENTS' SECTION IN THE OFFICE CONSENT BOOKLET AND THE PERSONAL CONSENT BOOKLET
CIRCLE CONSENT CODE 9 AT QUESTION 9 ON FRONT OF OFFICE CONSENT BOOKLET.
Press <1> and <Enter> to continue.
1   Continue

IF (StrUrA = No) OR (StrUrC = No) THEN
Code10
NURSE: CIRCLE CONSENT CODE 10 (NO CONSENT FOR URINE STORAGE) AT QUESTION 9 ON FRONT OF THE OFFICE CONSENT BOOKLET.
PRESS <1> AND <ENTER> TO CONTINUE
1   Continue

Thanks
 NURSE: THANK THE RESPONDENT FOR THEIR CO-OPERATION AND REMIND THEM THAT THEIR £10 GIFT VOUCHERS WILL BE POSTED TO THEM FROM THE OFFICE.
NURSE: REMEMBER TO LEAVE THE PALE GREY £10 PROMISSORY NOTE WITH THE RESPONDENT.
PRESS <1> AND <ENTER> TO CONTINUE
1   Continue

BLOOD SAMPLE
FOR ALL RESPONDENTS WHO ARE NOT PREGNANT

ASK ALL RESPONDENTS AGED 4+ EXCEPT PREGNANT WOMEN
BlIntro
NURSE: NOW FOLLOWS THE **BLOOD SAMPLE** MODULE.
NURSE: EXPLAIN THE PURPOSE AND PROCEDURE OF THE FASTING BLOOD
SAMPLE. GIVE RESPONDENT RELEVANT LEAFLETS.
1   Continue

IF (Age < 4) THEN
NFBlInt
NURSE: NOW FOLLOWS THE **BLOOD SAMPLE** MODULE.
NURSE: EXPLAIN THE PURPOSE AND PROCEDURE OF THE FASTING BLOOD
SAMPLE. GIVE RESPONDENT RELEVANT LEAFLETS.
1   Continue

IF (AGE <=16) THEN
ClotB
May I just check, do/(does) you/(child's name) have a clotting or bleeding disorder or
are/(is) you/(he/she) currently on anti-coagulant drugs such as Warfarin?
(NURSE: Aspirin therapy is not a contraindication for blood sample.)
1   Yes
2   No

IF (AGE <=16) AND (ClotB = No) THEN
Fit
May I just check, have/(has) you/(child's name) ever had a fit (including epileptic fit,
convulsion, convulsion associated with high fever)?
1   Yes
2   No

IF (AGE >=16) THEN
ClotBA
May I just check, do you have a clotting or bleeding disorder or are you currently on anti-
coagulant drugs such as Warfarin? (NURSE: Aspirin therapy is not a contraindication for
blood sample.)
NOTE TO NURSE: CLOPIDOGREL, PERSANTIN, DIPYRIDAMOLE AND OTHER
ANTI-PLATELET DRUGS ARE NOT A CONTRAINDICATION FOR BLOOD SAMPLE
1   Yes
2   No

IF (Age >=16) AND (ClotB = No) THEN
FitA
May I just check, have you had a fit (including epileptic fit or convulsion,) in the last five
years?
1   Yes
2   No

IF (Age >= 16) AND (ClotB = No) AND (Fit = No) THEN
BSWill
Would you be willing to have a fasting blood sample taken?
NURSE: THE RESPONDENT SHOULD FAST FOR 8 HOURS. REMIND HIM/HER
THAT THEY SHOULD DRINK WATER AS NORMAL.

1	Yes	"Yes"
2	No	"No"
3	Unable	"Respondent unable to give a blood sample for reason other than refusal (please specify at next question)"

IF (Age < 16) AND (ClotB = No) AND (Fit = No) THEN
CBSConst
ASK PARENT
Are you willing for your child to have a blood sample taken?
CHILDREN AGED 4 AND OVER SHOULD PROVIDE A FASTING SAMPLE.

1	Yes	
2	No	
3	Unable	"Respondent unable to give a blood sample for reason other than refusal (please specify at next question)"

IF (BSWill = No) OR (CBSConst = No) THEN
RefBSC
NURSE: Record why blood sample refused.
CODE ALL THAT APPLY.

1	PrevDiff	"Previous difficulties with venepuncture"
2	Fear	"Dislike/fear of needles"
3	RecTest	"Respondent recently had blood test/health check"
4	Ill	"Refused because of current illness"
5	HIV	"Worried about HIV or AIDS"
6	NoPaed	"No paediatric phlebotomist available"
7	Parent	"Parent doesn't agree with it/thinks child too young"
8	Busy	"Too busy"
9	Time	"Time constraints (i.e. appointment timings not convenient)"
97	Other	"Other"

IF (RefBSC = Other) THEN
OthRefBS
NURSE: Give full details of other reason(s) for refusing blood sample.
: STRING [135]

UnReas
NURSE: Record why respondent unable to give a blood sample (i.e. reason other than refusal).
: STRING[100]

IF (Age >= 4) AND (BSWill = Yes) OR (CBConst = Yes) THEN
Diabetes
NURSE: HAS THE RESPONDENT TOLD YOU THAT THEY ARE DIABETIC AND
UNWILLING TO FAST?
IF RESPONDENT IS DIABETIC AND CONCERNED ABOUT FASTING, PRESS F9
FOR GUIDANCE ABOUT THE DIFFERENT MEASURES THAT A DIABETIC COULD
TAKE AND STILL GIVE A FASTING BLOOD SAMPLE.
CODE BELOW WHETHER RESPONDENT WILLING TO GIVE A FASTING BLOOD
SAMPLE.
Acceptable procedures according to medication:
···Respondents on oral hypoglycaemic medication should be able to fast without
complications.
···Respondents on a combination of nightime insulin and daytime tablets should also be
able to fast unless they are known to have low blood sugar levels first thing in the
morning. If they do have low blood sugar in the morning, they could still fast but should
reduce their nightime insulin by a small amount and have breakfast as soon as possible
after the blood is taken.
···Respondents on insulin alone can also provide a fasting sample, but should be given
special consideration. They should omit their morning insulin and should be seen as
early in the day as possible.
In every case, diabetics should have breakfast as soon as possible after blood is taken.
**Note that the option of providing a non-fasting sample is only open to diabetics
and respondents under the age of 4. Blood should not be taken from respondents
who are willing to provide a sample but are not prepared to fast.**
1   NotDiab   "Not diabetic/not mentioned"
2   Yes   "Diabetic and willing to give fasting blood"
3   No   "Diabetic and not willing to give fasting blood sample"

IF (Diabetes = No) THEN
DiabNF
NURSE: THIS PERSON SHOULD GIVE A NON-FASTING BLOOD SAMPLE. THIS
BLOOD SAMPLE SHOULD BE TAKEN AT THE SAME TIME AS A FASTING BLOOD
SAMPLE FROM OTHER HOUSEHOLD MEMBERS (IF APPLICABLE).
1   Continue

IF (Diabetes = NotDiab OR Yes) THEN
IsTime
NURSE: IS THE TIME CURRENTLY BEFORE 10 AM?
1   Yes
2   No

IF (IsTime = Yes) AND (Computer time = before 10am) THEN
Eat
Can I check, have you had anything to eat or drink (excluding water) in the last 8 hours?
1   Yes
2   No

IF (Diabetes = No) OR ((Age < 11) AND (Nurse = paediatric phlebotomist)) THEN
NFastBl
NURSE: THIS RESPONDENT COULD GIVE A NON-FASTING BLOOD SAMPLE NOW.
BEFORE DECIDING WHETHER TO TAKE BLOOD, CHECK:

Are the labs open (i.e. is it Monday - Thursday)/expecting a sample?
Is there anyone else in the household who will give blood?
If so, could you take blood from both respondents at the same time (i.e. a return visit)?
CONSIDER THESE QUESTIONS AND CODE:
1   Yes   Yes, I will take the blood sample now
2   No   No, I will return at a later date to take the blood sample

IF (NFastBl = No) THEN
NFSAppt
NURSE: ARRANGE AN APPOINTMENT WITH (respondent's name) TO TAKE A
BLOOD SAMPLE. THIS SHOULD BE ON A MONDAY TO THURSDAY MORNING
ONLY
1   Continue

IF (Eat = No) THEN
FastBl
NURSE: THIS RESPONDENT COULD GIVE A FASTING BLOOD SAMPLE NOW.
BEFORE DECIDING WHETHER TO TAKE BLOOD, CHECK:
IF CHILD UNDER 4: ARE YOU A TRAINED PAEDIATRIC PHLEBOTOMIST? (IF NO,
CODE 2)
Are the labs open/expecting a sample?
Is there anyone else in the household who will give blood?
If so, you should take blood from both respondents at the same time.
CONSIDER THESE QUESTIONS AND CODE:
1   Yes   "Yes, I will take the fasting blood sample now"
2   No   "No, I will return at a later date to take the blood sample"

IF (FastBl = No) THEN
FBAppt
NURSE: ARRANGE AN APPOINTMENT WITH (respondent's name) TO TAKE A
BLOOD SAMPLE. THIS SHOULD BE BEFORE 10AM, MONDAY TO THURSDAY
ONLY
1   Continue

IF (Age <= 16) THEN
AmeInt
NURSE: Explain that there is the option of using Ametop gel, but that a sample can be
given without Ametop.
Give parent/respondent the Ametop information sheet and allow them time to read it.
Ask respondent/parent whether they think they will want to use Ametop. If they do, you
need to schedule your return appointment before 9.30am.
1   Continue

IF BLOOD SAMPLE NOT TAKEN ON FIRST VISIT THEN
IntFBT
NURSE: NOW FOLLOWS THE MODULE TO OBTAIN BLOOD SAMPLES.
1   Continue

IF (AGE <16) THEN
TClotB
May I just check again, do/(does) you/(child's name)have a clotting or bleeding disorder or are you currently on anti-coagulant drugs such as Warfarin?
(NURSE: Aspirin therapy is not a contraindication for blood sample.)
1   Yes
2   No

IF (TClotB=No) THEN
TFit
May I just check also, have/(has) you/(child's name) ever had a fit (including epileptic fit, convulsion, convulsion associated with high fever)?
1   Yes
2   No

IF (AGE > 16) THEN
TClotBA
May I just check, do you have a clotting or bleeding disorder or are you currently on anti-coagulant drugs such as Warfarin?
NURSE: Aspirin therapy is not a contraindication for blood sample
NOTE TO NURSE: CLOPIDOGREL, PERSANTIN, DIPYRIDAMOLE AND OTHER ANTI-PLATELET DRUGS ARE NOT A CONTRAINDICATION FOR BLOOD SAMPLE.
1   Yes
2   No

IF (AGE > 16) THEN
TFitA
May I just check, have you had a fit (including epileptic fit or convulsion,) in the last five years?
1   Yes
2   No

IF (TFitC = No) AND (Age >=4) THEN
TEat
Can I check, have you had anything to eat or drink (excluding water) in the last 8 hours?
1   Yes
2   No

IF (TFitC = No) AND (Age <4) THEN
ChEat
Can I check, has (respondent's name) had anything to eat or drink (excluding water) in the last 8 hours?
1   Yes
2   No

IF (TEat = Yes) OR (ChEat = Yes) THEN
ReArr
NURSE: The respondent has eaten something and cannot give a fasting blood sample today. Try to rearrange the appointment for another day.
1   Appt   "Appointment rearranged to take blood"
2   NoAppt   "Not able to make another appointment"

IF (2nd visit AND ReArr = NoAppt) OR (3rd visit) THEN

IF (2nd visit AND ReArr = NoAppt) OR (3rd visit) THEN
TBSStop
No Blood Samples should be taken from ^PName. Ring codes 12,14, 16, 18 on the consent booklet
1   Continue

IF (2nd visit AND ReArr = Appt) THEN
TBSNoV2
No Blood Samples should be taken from (respondent's name) now. You will need to make another visit to take blood.
1   Continue

IF (Age >= 16) THEN
TBSWill
Would you be willing to have a fasting/(non-fasting) blood sample taken?
1   Yes
2   No
3   Unable   "Respondent unable to give a blood for reason other than refusal (please specify at next question)"

IF (Age < 16) THEN
TCBSConst
ASK PARENT
Are you willing for your child to have a fasting/(non-fasting) blood sample taken?
NURSE: CHECK THAT CHILD IS WILLING ALSO, EXPLAIN PROCESS AND REASSURE THEM. ONLY TRAINED PAEDIATRIC PHLEBOTOMISTS SHOULD TAKE BLOOD FROM CHILDREN UNDER 11.
1   Yes
2   No
3   Unable   "Respondent unable to give a blood for reason other than refusal (please specify at next question)"

IF (TCBSConst = Yes) THEN
AmetopUse
(ASK PARENT)
Do you want Ametop gel to be used?
1   Yes
2   No

IF (AmetopUse = Yes) THEN
Allergy
(ASK PARENT)
Have/(Has) you/(he/she) ever had a bad reaction to a local or general anaesthetic bought over the counter at a chemist, or given at the doctor, the dentist or in hospital?
1   Yes
2   No

IF (Allergy = Yes) THEN
NoAmetop
NURSE: Ametop gel cannot be used. Is respondent willing to give blood sample without Ametop gel?
Code 1 if Yes, willing to give blood sample without Ametop gel
Code 2 if No, not willing to give blood sample without Ametop
1   Yes   "Yes, willing"
2   No   "No, no blood sample"
IF (Allergy = No) THEN
DoAmetop
NURSE: **Blood sample with Ametop gel**.
- Check you have all applicable signatures.
- Apply Ametop gel following instructions.
- Wait at least half an hour before attempting blood sample.
1   Continue

IF (BSWill = No) OR (CBSConst = No) THEN
TRefBSC
NURSE: Record why blood sample refused.
CODE ALL THAT APPLY.
PrevDiff   "Previous difficulties with venepuncture",
Fear   "Dislike/fear of needles",
RecTest   "Respondent recently had blood test/health check",
Ill   "Refused because of current illness",
HIV   "Worried about HIV or AIDS",
NoPaed   "No paediatric phlebotomist available",
Parent   "Parent doesn't agree with it/thinks child too young",
Busy   "Too busy",
Time   "Time constraints (i.e. appointment timings not convenient)",
Other   "Other"

TOthRef
NURSE: Give full details of other reason(s) for refusing blood sample.
: STRING [135]

TUnReas
NURSE: Record why respondent unable to give a blood sample (i.e. reason other than refusal).
: STRING [100]

IF (TBSWill = Yes) OR ((TCBSConst = Yes) AND (AmetopUse = No)) OR ((TCBSConst = Yes) AND (AmetopUse = Yes) AND (Allergy = No)) OR ((TCBSConst = Yes) AND (AmetopUse = Yes) AND (Allergy = Yes) AND (NoAmetop = Yes)) THEN
BSConsC
NURSE: Explain need for written consent from parent:
Before I can take any blood, I have to obtain the written consent from both parent and child/(written consent from you).
1   Continue

IF (Age = 18 months - 15) THEN
GuardCon
NURSE CHECK: Is a parent or person with legal responsibility willing to give consent?
1   Yes
2   No

IF (GuardCon = No) THEN
Ignore
NURSE: Record details of why consent refused.
: STRING [140]

Code11C
NURSE:
- ASK PARENT/LEGAL GUARDIAN TO INITIAL FIRST BOX IN 'BLOOD SAMPLING CONSENTS' SECTION IN THE OFFICE CONSENT BOOKLET AND THE PERSONAL CONSENT BOOKLET.
- MAKE SURE *(child's)* NAME IS FILLED IN BOTH COPIES.
- ASK PARENT/LEGAL GUARDIAN TO SIGN AND DATE AT THE BOTTOM OF THE PAGE IN BOTH COPIES.
- TICK THE BOX "With the use of Ametop"
- CIRCLE CONSENT CODE 11 AT QUESTION 9 ON FRONT OF THE OFFICE CONSENT BOOKLET.
Press <1> and <Enter> to continue.
1   Continue

Code11A
NURSE:
- ASK RESPONDENT TO INITIAL FIRST BOX IN 'BLOOD SAMPLING CONSENTS' SECTION IN THE OFFICE CONSENT BOOKLET AND THE PERSONAL CONSENT BOOKLET.
- MAKE SURE RESPONDENT'S NAME IS FILLED IN BOTH COPIES.
- ASK RESPONDENT TO SIGN AND DATE AT THE BOTTOM OF THE PAGE IN BOTH COPIES.
- CIRCLE CONSENT CODE 11 AT QUESTION 9 ON FRONT OF THE OFFICE CONSENT BOOKLET.
Press <1> and <Enter> to continue.
1   Continue

IF (TBSStop=1) THEN
Code12
NURSE: CIRCLE CONSENT CODE 12 (NO CONSENT FOR BLOOD SAMPLING) AT QUESTION 9 ON FRONT OF THE OFFICE CONSENT BOOKLET.

Press <1> and <Enter> to continue.
1   Continue

IF (GPRegBP <> Yes) OR (GPRegBM <> Yes) OR (Age = 18 months – 3) THEN
GPRegFB
NURSE CHECK: Is respondent registered with a GP?
1   Yes   "Respondent registered with GP"
2   No   "Respondent not registered with GP"

IF (GPRegFB = Yes) THEN
SendSam
May we send the results of your/(child's name)'s blood sample analysis to your/(his/her) GP?
1   Yes
2   No

IF (SendSam = Yes) THEN
Code13
"NURSE:
- Obtain initials and signature in **both** the Consent Booklet and the Respondent Copy.
- Check name by which GP knows respondent.
- Check GP name, address and phone no. are recorded on front of the Consent Booklet.
- Circle consent **code 13** on front of the Consent Booklet.
1   Continue

IF (SendSam = No) THEN
SenSaC
Why do you not want your/(child's name)'s blood sample results sent to your/(his/her) GP?
1   NeverSee   "Hardly/never sees GP"
2   RecSamp   "GP recently took blood sample"
3   Bother   "Does not want to bother GP"
4   Other   "Other"

IF (SenSaC = Other) THEN
OthSam
NURSE: Give full details of reason(s) for not wanting results sent to GP.
: STRING [140]

IF (SendSam = No) THEN
Code14
NURSE: Circle consent **code 14** on front of the Consent Booklet.
1   Continue

SnDrSam
Would you like to be sent the results of your/(child's name)'s blood sample analysis?
1   Yes
2   No

IF (SnDrSam = Yes) THEN

NDNS YEAR 3 CAPI_NURSE

Code17
NURSE: Circle consent **code 17** on front of the Consent Booklet.
1	Continue

IF (SnDrSam = No) THEN
Code18
NURSE: Circle consent **code 18** on front of the Consent Booklet.
1	Continue

IF (SendSam = No) AND (SnDrSam = No) THEN
GPDisc
NURSE: THIS RESPONDENT DOES NOT WANT THEIR RESULTS SENT TO THEIR
GP. PLEASE ASK THEM TO READ AND SIGN THE DISCLAIMER IN THE
RESPONDENT AND OFFICE CONSENT BOOKLETS.
1	Continue

IF (TBSWill = Yes) THEN
ConStorB
ASK Respondent: May we have your consent to store any remaining blood for future
analysis?
NURSE: IF ASKED, 'THE BLOOD WOULD BE USED FOR TESTS RELATING TO
NUTRITION AND HEALTH. THE TESTS WOULD BE APPROVED BY AN ETHICS
COMMITTEE'. NURSE: IF ASKED, EXPLAIN THE RESPONDENT CAN WITHDRAW
THEIR CONSENT AT ANY TIME, WITHOUT GIVING ANY REASON, BY ASKING THE
INVESTIGATORS IN WRITING FOR BLOOD TO BE REMOVED FROM STORAGE
AND DESTROYED.
1	Yes	"Storage consent given",
2	No	"Consent refused"), NODK, NORF

IF (ConStorB = Yes) THEN
Code15
NURSE:
- Obtain initials and signatures in **both** the Consent Booklet and the Respondent Copy.
- Circle consent **code 15** on front of the Consent Booklet.
1	Continue

IF (ConStorB = No) THEN
Code16
NURSE: Circle consent **code 16** on front of the Consent Booklet.
1	Continue

IF (Age >= 16) THEN
TakeSAd
NURSE: First check you have **all applicable signatures**, then:
A) Take blood samples in the following order:
·····1. EDTA (2.6ml) tube **red** cap, label E N1 (3)
·····2. serum (4.5ml) tube **brown** cap, label SE N1 (5)
·····3. serum (4.5ml) tube **white** cap, label SE N2 (6)
·····4. Lithium heparin (7.5ml) tube **orange** cap, label LH N1 (7)
·····5. Lithium heparin (7.5ml) tube **orange** cap, label LH N2 (8)
·····6. Fluoride (1.2 ml) tube **yellow** cap, label F N1 (10)

·····7. Lithium/heparin (4.5ml) tube **orange** cap, label LH N3 (9)
·····8. EDTA (2.7ml) tube **red** cap, label E N2 (4)
B) Check the date of birth again with the respondent to ensure you have the right labels for the right respondent
C) Stick the barcoded label HORIZONTALLY over the label which is already on the tube.
D) Stick appropriate barcoded label on the field lab and Addenbrookes despatch notes.
E) Remember to attach labels FOL 1 (37) and FOL 2 (38) to the 3 carbonised
copies of the completed Addenbrookes biochemistry despatch note using a paper clip.
- Check to ensure you have used the correct barcoded labels for THIS
respondent····Serial number: *(displayed)*
PLEASE REMEMBER TO DELIVER A PACK OF MICRO-TUBES (ADULT AGED 16+)
TO YOUR LOCAL LAB WHEN YOU DELIVER THESE SAMPLES!
1   Continue

SampF1A
NURSE: Code if the 1st EDTA (red, 2.6ml) tube filled (label E N1 (3)).
1   YesF   "Yes, FULLY filled"
2   YesP   "Yes, PARTIALLY filled"
3   No   "No, not filled"

IF (Age >= 16) THEN
SampF2A
NURSE: Code if the 1st serum (brown, 4.7ml) tube filled (label SE N1 (5)).
1   YesF   "Yes, FULLY filled"
2   YesP   "Yes, PARTIALLY filled"
3   No   "No, not filled"

IF (Age >= 16) THEN
SampF3A
NURSE: Code if the 2nd serum (white, 4.5ml) tube filled (label SE N2 (6)).
1   YesF   "Yes, FULLY filled"
2   YesP   "Yes, PARTIALLY filled"
3   No   "No, not filled"

IF (Age >= 16) THEN
SampF4A
NURSE: Code if the 1st Lithium/heparin (orange, 7.5ml) tube filled (label LH N1 (7)).
1   YesF   "Yes, FULLY filled"
2   YesP   "Yes, PARTIALLY filled"
3   No   "No, not filled"

IF (Age >= 16) THEN
SampF5A
NURSE: Code if the 2nd Lithium heparin (orange, 7.5ml) tube filled (label LH N2 (8)).
1   YesF   "Yes, FULLY filled"
2   YesP   "Yes, PARTIALLY filled"
3   No   "No, not filled"

IF (Age >= 16) THEN
SampF6A
NURSE: Code if the fluoride (yellow, 1.2ml) tube filled (label F N1 (10)).

1	YesF	"Yes, FULLY filled"
2	YesP	"Yes, PARTIALLY filled"
3	No	"No, not filled"

IF (Age >= 16) THEN
SampF7A
NURSE: Code if 3rd lithuim heparin (orange, 4.5 ml) tube filled (label LH N3 (9)).

1	YesF	"Yes, FULLY filled"
2	YesP	"Yes, PARTIALLY filled"
3	No	"No, not filled"

IF (Age >= 16) THEN
SampF8A
NURSE: Code if 2nd EDTA (red, 2.6ml) tube filled (label E N2 (4)).

1	YesF	"Yes, FULLY filled"
2	YesP	"Yes, PARTIALLY filled"
3	No	"No, not filled"

IF (Age = 7 – 15) THEN
TakeSCO
NURSE: First check you have **all applicable signatures**, then:
A) Take blood samples in the following order:
·····1. EDTA (2.6ml) tube **red** cap, label E N1 (3)
·····2. Lithium heparin (7.5ml) tube **orange** cap, label LH N1 (7)
·····3. Serum (2.7ml) tube **brown** cap, label SE N1 (5)
·····4. Serum (2.7ml) tube **white** cap, label SE N2 (6)
·····5. Lithium heparin (2.7ml) tube **orange** cap, label LH N2 (8)
·····6. Fluoride (1.2 ml) tube **yellow** cap, label F N1 (10)
B) Check the date of birth again with the respondent to ensure you have the right labels for the right respondent
C) Stick the barcoded label HORIZONTALLY over the label which is already on the tube.
D) Stick appropriate barcoded label on the field lab and Addenbrookes despatch notes.
E) Remember to attach labels FOL 1 (37) and FOL 2 (38) to the 3 carbonised
copies of the completed Addenbrookes biochemistry despatch note using a paper clip.
- Check to ensure you have used the correct barcoded labels for THIS
respondent····Serial number: *(displayed)*
PLEASE REMEMBER TO DELIVER A PACK OF MICRO-TUBES (CHILD AGED 7-15)
TO YOUR LOCAL LAB WHEN YOU DELIVER THESE SAMPLES!

| 1 | Continue |

IF (Age = 7 – 15) THEN
SampF1CO
NURSE: Code if the EDTA (red, 2.6ml) tube filled (label E N1 (3)).

1	YesF	"Yes, FULLY filled"
2	YesP	"Yes, PARTIALLY filled"
3	No	"No, not filled"

IF (Age = 7 – 15) THEN
SampF2CO
NURSE: Code if the 1st lithium heparin (orange, 7.5ml) tube filled (label LH N1 (7))

| 1 | YesF | "Yes, FULLY filled" |

| 2 | YesP | "Yes, PARTIALLY filled" |
| 3 | No | "No, not filled" |

IF (Age = 7 – 15) THEN
SampF3CO
NURSE: Code if the 1st serum (brown, 2.6ml) tube filled (label SE N1 (5)).

1	YesF	"Yes, FULLY filled"
2	YesP	"Yes, PARTIALLY filled"
3	No	"No, not filled"

IF (Age = 7 – 15) THEN
SampF4CO
NURSE: Code if the 2nd serum (white, 4.5ml) tube filled (label SE N2 (6)).

1	YesF	"Yes, FULLY filled"
2	YesP	"Yes, PARTIALLY filled"
3	No	"No, not filled"

IF (Age = 7 – 15) THEN
SampF5CO
NURSE: Code if the 2nd lithium heparin (orange, 2.7ml) tube filled (label LH N2 (8))."

1	YesF	"Yes, FULLY filled"
2	YesP	"Yes, PARTIALLY filled"
3	No	"No, not filled"

IF (Age = 7 – 15) THEN
SampF6CO
NURSE: Code if Fluoride (yellow, 1.2ml) tube filled (label F N1 (10)).

1	YesF	"Yes, FULLY filled"
2	YesP	"Yes, PARTIALLY filled"
3	No	"No, not filled"

IF (Age = 18 months - 6) THEN
TakeSCY
NURSE: First check you have **all applicable signatures**, then:
A) Take blood samples in the following order:
·····1. EDTA (2.6ml) tube **red** cap, label EN1 (3)
·····2. Lithium/heparin (4.5ml) tube **orange** cap, label LH N1 (7)
·····3. Serum (1.2ml) tube **brown** cap, label SE N1 (5)
·····4. Serum (2.7ml) tube **white** cap, label SE N2 (6)
B) Check the date of birth again with the respondent to ensure you have the right labels for the right respondent
C) Stick the barcoded label HORIZONTALLY over the label which is already on the tube.
D) Stick appropriate barcoded label on the field lab and Addenbrookes despatch notes.
E) Remember to attach labels FOL 1 (37) and FOL 2 (38) to the 3 carbonised
copies of the completed Addenbrookes biochemistry despatch note using a paper clip.
- Check to ensure you have used the correct barcoded labels for this respondent····Serial number: *(displayed)*
PLEASE REMEMBER TO DELIVER A PACK OF MICRO-TUBES (CHILD AGED 18mths-6yrs) TO YOUR LOCAL LAB WHEN YOU DELIVER THESE SAMPLES!

| 1 | Continue |

IF (Age = 18 months - 6) THEN
SampF1CY
NURSE: Code if the EDTA (red, 2.6ml) tube filled (label E N1 (3)).
1   YesF   "Yes, FULLY filled"
2   YesP   "Yes, PARTIALLY filled"
3   No   "No, not filled"

IF (Age = 18 months - 6) THEN
SampF2CY
NURSE: Code if the Lithium heparin (orange, 4.5ml) tube filled (label LH N1 (7)).
1   YesF   "Yes, FULLY filled"
2   YesP   "Yes, PARTIALLY filled"
3   No   "No, not filled"

IF (Age = 18 months - 6) THEN
SampF3CY
NURSE: Code if the 1st serum (brown, 1.1ml) tube filled (label SE N1 (5)).
1   YesF   "Yes, FULLY filled"
2   YesP   "Yes, PARTIALLY filled"
3   No   "No, not filled"

IF (Age = 18 months - 6) THEN
SampF4CY
NURSE: Code if the 2nd serum (white, 2.7ml) tube filled (label SE N2 (6)).
1   YesF   "Yes, FULLY filled"
2   YesP   "Yes, PARTIALLY filled"
3   No   "No, not filled"

SampTak
Blood sample outcome *(COMPUTED)*:
1   YesF   "Blood sample obtained - all full"
2   YesP   "Blood sample obtained - not all full"
3   No   "No blood sample obtained"

IF (SampTak = YesF OR YesP) THEN
SamDifC
NURSE: Record any problems in taking blood sample.
CODE ALL THAT APPLY.
1   NoProb   "No problem"
2   Small   "Incomplete sample"
3   BadVein   "Collapsing/poor veins"
4   TakeTwo   "Second attempt necessary"
5   Faint   "Some blood obtained, but respondent felt faint/fainted"
6   NoTour   "Unable to use tourniquet"
7   Other   "Other (SPECIFY AT NEXT QUESTION)

IF (SamDifC = Other) THEN
OthBDif
NURSE: Give full details of other problem(s) in taking blood sample.

: STRING [140]

IF (SampTak = No) THEN
NoBSC
NURSE: Code reason(s) why no blood obtained.
CODE ALL THAT APPLY.

1	NoVein	"No suitable or no palpable vein/collapsed veins"
2	Anxious	"Respondent was too anxious/nervous"
3	Faint	"Respondent felt faint/fainted"
4	Other (97)	"Other"

IF (NoBSC = Other) THEN
OthNoBSM
NURSE: Give full details of reason(s) no blood obtained.

IF (SampTak = No) THEN
Code10
NURSE:
- Cross out consent codes **11, 13, 15 and 17** if already circled on front of the Consent Booklet.
- Replace with consent codes **12, 14, 16 and 18** on front of the Consent Booklet.
1   Continue

ThanksB
NURSE: THANK THE RESPONDENT FOR THEIR CO-OPERATION AND REMIND THEM THAT THEIR £15 GIFT VOUCHERS WILL BE POSTED TO THEM FROM THE OFFICE.
NURSE: REMEMBER TO LEAVE THE YELLOW £15 PROMISSORY NOTE WITH THE RESPONDENT.
1   Continue

DRUGS

DrC1
NURSE : Enter code for (*drug*).
 : STRING [6]

YTake1
Do you take (*drug*) because of a heart problem, high blood pressure or for some other reason?
Heart   "Heart problem",
HBP   "High blood pressure",
Other   "Other reason"

TakeOth1
NURSE : Give full details of reason(s) for taking (*drug*).
Press <Esc> when finished.
 : OPEN

SERIAL NUMBER (7 DIGITS)   CKL   PERSON NO.

NDNS NHS (A)

National Diet and Nutrition Survey (NDNS)

NHS Central Register and Cancer Register

(Adults 16+)

- The NHS Central Register lists all the people in the country and their National Health Service (NHS) number.

- We would like to ask for your consent for us to send your name, address and date of birth to the National Health Service Central Register. A marker will be put against your name to show that you took part in the National Diet and Nutrition Survey.

- If a person who took part in the National Diet and Nutrition Survey gets cancer, or dies, the type of cancer or cause of death will be linked with their answers to the survey. By linking this information the research is more useful as we can look at how people's lifestyle can have an impact on their future health.

- This information will be confidential and used for research purposes only.

- By signing this form you are only giving permission for the linking of this information to routine administrative data and nothing else. We will not be able to obtain any other details from your medical records.

- You can cancel this permission at any time in the future by writing to us at the following address:

    National Centre for Social Research, 35 Northampton Square, London EC1V 0AX

Your consent

I, (name) _____ consent to the NDNS team passing my name, address and date of birth to the **National Health Service Central Register**. I understand that information held by **the NHS Central Register** may be used to follow up my health status.

Signed _____   *Date* _____

I understand that these details will be used for research purposes only.

National Diet and Nutrition Survey (NDNS)

CONSENT BOOKLET: PERSONAL COPY

Serial Number:

First Name:

CONSENT FORM FOR NDNS

ADULT AGED 16+

Respondent's name_____(BLOCK LETTERS)

- I have received the information leaflets (Interviewer and Nurse versions) which explain the nature and purpose of the study. I have read and understood these leaflets.
- I am satisfied with any enquiries I have made regarding the study.
- I have been informed that the results will be kept confidential and presented in a way that protects my identity.
- I understand that I may withdraw my consent to any or all of the survey elements at any time without needing to give a reason.

I hereby consent to the following aspects of the study:

BLOOD PRESSURE (TO GP) CONSENT:
Please initial box if consent given

[ ] The survey team sending my blood pressure measurement to my GP.

BMI (TO GP) CONSENT:
Please initial box if consent given

[ ] The survey team sending my body mass index (BMI) measurements to my GP.

24 HOUR URINE CONSENTS:
Please initial box if consent given

[ ] Taking PABA tablets to support the 24-hour urine collection.

[ ] Laboratory analysis of my 24-hour urine collection, to help assess my diet.

[ ] Storage of any remaining urine for tests in the future relating to nutrition and health, provided that the tests are approved by an NHS ethics committee. I understand that I can withdraw my consent to store my urine at any time, without giving any reason, by asking the investigators in writing for my urine to be removed from storage and destroyed. I understand that my data is being used in anonymised form only.

Signature: ....Date ....

CONSENT FORM FOR NDNS

CF (A2)

ADULT AGED 16+

Respondent's name_____(BLOCK LETTERS)

- I have received the information leaflets (Interviewer and Nurse versions) which explain the nature and purpose of the study. I have read and understood these leaflets.

- I am satisfied with any enquiries I have made regarding the study.

- I have been informed that the results will be kept confidential and presented in a way that protects my identity.

- I understand that I may withdraw my consent to any or all of the survey elements at any time without needing to give a reason.

I hereby consent to the following aspects of the study:

BLOOD SAMPLING CONSENTS:

Please initial box if consent given

☐ Having a blood sample for tests related to nutrition and health. This blood sample will not be used for HIV or genetic testing.

☐ I would like / would not like *(delete as appropriate)* to receive a written report of my clinically relevant blood results*.

☐ The NDNS team sending my potentially clinically relevant blood results to my GP*.

☐ Storage of any remaining blood for tests in the future relating to nutrition and health, provided that the tests are approved by an NHS ethics committee. I understand that I can withdraw my consent to store my blood at any time, without giving any reason, by asking the investigators in writing for my blood to be removed from storage and destroyed. I understand that my data is being used in anonymised form only.

*Please note that if you do not want to receive a report of your blood results **and** do not want results to be passed on to your GP we need you to sign a disclaimer (page 6).

Signature: ……………………………………………………Date ……………………….

CONSENT FORM FOR NDNS

CHILDREN AGED 4 TO 15 YEARS

Parent/Guardian Section

I agree for my child to participate in the above named survey and in doing so acknowledge that:

- I have received the information leaflets (Interviewer and Nurse versions) which explain the nature and purpose of the study. I have read and understood these leaflets.

- I am satisfied with any enquiries I have made regarding the study.

- I have been informed that the results will be kept confidential and presented in a way that protects my child's identity.

- I understand that I may withdraw my consent to any or all of the survey elements at any time without needing to give a reason.

I hereby agree for my child to participate in the following aspects of the survey:

BLOOD PRESSURE (TO GP) CONSENT:

Please initial box if consent given

☐ The survey team sending his/her blood pressure measurement to his/her GP.

24 HOUR URINE CONSENTS:

Please initial box if consent given

☐ Taking PABA tablets to support the 24-hour urine collection.

☐ Laboratory analysis of his/her 24-hour urine collection, to help assess his/her diet.

☐ Storage of any remaining urine for tests in the future relating to nutrition and health, provided that the tests are approved by an NHS ethics committee. I understand that I can withdraw my consent to store my child's urine at any time, without giving any reason, by asking the investigators in writing for his/her urine to be removed from storage and destroyed. I understand that my data is being used in anonymised form only.

Respondent's (Child's) Name:...

Parent/Guardian Name: ....

Parent/Guardian signature: ....Date ....

Child assent

I agree to take part in the NDNS survey. I understand the measurements that will be made.

Respondent (Child) signature: ....Date...........................

CONSENT FORM FOR NDNS

CHILDREN AGED 4 TO 15 YEARS

Parent/Guardian Section

I agree for my child to participate in the above named survey and in doing so acknowledge that:

- I have received the information leaflets (Interviewer and Nurse versions) which explain the nature and purpose of the study. I have read and understood these leaflets.

- I am satisfied with any enquiries I have made regarding the study.

- I have been informed that the results will be kept confidential and presented in a way that protects my child's identity.

- I understand that I may withdraw my consent to any or all of the survey elements at any time without needing to give a reason.

- I have been given written information about the Ametop gel and the nurse has explained the purpose and use of Ametop gel to me.

I hereby agree for my child to participate in the following aspects of the survey:

BLOOD SAMPLING CONSENTS:

Please initial box if consent given

☐	Blood sample for tests related to nutrition and health. This blood sample will not be used for HIV or genetic testing. Please tick the appropriate box:

    ☐ with Ametop gel   ☐ without Ametop gel

☐	I would like / would not like *(delete as appropriate)* to receive a written report of my child's clinically relevant blood results*.
☐	The NDNS team sending potentially clinically relevant blood results to his/her GP*.
☐	Storage of any remaining blood for tests in the future relating to nutrition and health, provided that the tests are approved by an NHS ethics committee. I understand that I can withdraw my consent to store my child's blood at any time, without giving any reason, by asking the investigators in writing for his/her blood to be removed from storage and destroyed. I understand that my data is being used in anonymised form only.

*Please note that if you do not want to receive a report of your child's blood results **and** do not want results to be passed on to his/her GP we need you to sign a disclaimer (page 6).

Respondent's (Child's) Name:...

Parent/Guardian Name: ....

Parent/Guardian signature: ....Date ....

Child assent

I agree to take part in the NDNS survey. I understand the measurements that will be made.

Respondent (Child) signature: ....Date.........................

CONSENT FORM FOR NDNS

CHILDREN AGED 1.5 TO 3 YEARS

Parent/Guardian Section

I agree for my child to participate in the above named survey and in doing so acknowledge that:

- I have received the information leaflets (Interviewer and Nurse versions) which explain the nature and purpose of the study. I have read and understood these leaflets.

- I am satisfied with any enquiries I have made regarding the study.

- I have been informed that the results will be kept confidential and presented in a way that protects my child's identity.

- I understand that I may withdraw my consent to any or all of the study elements at any time without needing to give a reason.

- I have been given written information about the Ametop gel and the nurse has explained the purpose and use of Ametop gel to me.

I hereby agree for my child to participate in the following aspects of the study:

BLOOD SAMPLING CONSENTS:

Please initial box if consent given

☐ Blood sample for tests related to nutrition and health. This blood sample will not be used for HIV or genetic testing. Please tick the appropriate box:

　　☐ with Ametop gel　　　　☐ without Ametop gel

☐ I would like / would not like *(delete as appropriate)* to receive a written report of my child's clinically relevant blood results*.

☐ The NDNS team sending potentially clinically relevant blood results to his/her GP*.

☐ Storage of any remaining blood for tests in the future relating to nutrition and health, provided that the tests are approved by an NHS ethics committee. I understand that I can withdraw my consent to store my child's blood at any time, without giving any reason, by asking the investigators in writing for his/her blood to be removed from storage and destroyed. I understand that my data is being used in anonymised form only.

*Please note that if you do not want to receive a report of his/her blood results **and** do not want results to be passed on to his/her GP we need you to sign a disclaimer (page 6).

Respondent's (Child's) Name:..

Parent/Guardian Name: ....

Parent/Guardian signature: ....Date ....

NDNS DISCLAIMER

Date:........................

Name:.. (Block letters)

Respondent's name: .... (Block letters)
(if different from above)

This is to clarify that against the advice of the NDNS survey team I:

Please initial boxes

☐ Do not want to receive <u>my</u> / <u>my child's</u> *(delete as appropriate)* clinically relevant examination results

☐ Do not want <u>my</u> / <u>my child's</u> *(delete as appropriate)* clinically relevant examination results being sent to <u>my</u> / <u>his/her</u> *(delete as appropriate)* GP

I do understand that if there are findings outside the normal range this will not be brought to the attention of any health care provider.

By doing so, I assume all responsibility for my act.

Signed:..

Nurse:..

National Diet and Nutrition Survey – Consent Booklet: Office Copy

Please use capital letters and write in ink

ADDRESS

INDIVIDUAL SERIAL NUMBER:
Affix label **NCON** here for this person:

STICK *NCON* (1) LABEL HERE

1. Nurse number: ☐☐☐☐ ☐☐

2. Date schedule completed (all visits complete): DAY ☐☐ MONTH ☐☐ YEAR ☐☐☐☐

3. Full name (of person tested) _____

   Name by which GP knows person (if different) _____

4. Sex   Male ☐ 1   Female ☐ 2

5. Date of birth: DAY ☐☐ MONTH ☐☐ YEAR ☐☐☐☐

6. Full name of parent/guardian (*if person under 16*) _____

7.
GP NAME AND ADDRESS
Dr: ....
Practice Name: ....
Address: ....
....
Town: ....
County: ....
Postcode: ....
Telephone no: ....

8. **NURSE USE ONLY**

GP Address complete	1
GP Address not complete	2
No GP	3

9.

SUMMARY OF CONSENTS - RING CODE FOR EACH ITEM	YES	NO
a) Blood pressure to **GP**	01	02
b) Body Mass Index (BMI) to **GP**	03	04
c) Take PABA tablet	05	06
d) Lab analysis of Urine	07	08
e) Urine sample for **storage**	09	10
f) Sample of blood to be taken	11	12
g) Blood sample result to **GP**	13	14
h) Blood sample for **storage**	15	16
i) Blood sample result to **respondent**	17	18

BLOOD SAMPLE LABORATORY REFERENCE LIST

The tables below show which blood samples should be taken (in priority order) and need to be sent to each lab for each age group:

RESPONDENTS AGED 16+

Priority	Blood Tube	Colour	Label Reference	Laboratory	Despatch note
1	EDTA 1	RED	E N1	Addenbrookes	DESP ADDX
2	SERUM 1	BROWN	SE N1	Addenbrookes	DESP ADDX
3	SERUM 2	WHITE	SE N2	Field Lab	DESP FL2.1
4	LI HEP 1	ORANGE	LH N1	Field Lab	DESP FL2.1
5	LI HEP 2	ORANGE	LH N2	Field Lab	DESP FL2.1
6	FLUORIDE	YELLOW	F N1	Field Lab	DESP FL2.1
7	LI HEP 3	ORANGE	LH N3	Field Lab	DESP FL2.1
8	EDTA 2	RED	E N2	Field Lab	DESP FL2.1

RESPONDENTS AGED 7-15

Priority	Blood Tube	Colour	Label Reference	Laboratory	Despatch note
1	EDTA 1	RED	E N1	Addenbrookes	DESP ADDX
2	LI HEP 1	ORANGE	LH N1	Field Lab	DESP FL2.2
3	SERUM 1	BROWN	SE N1	Addenbrookes	DESP ADDX
4	SERUM 2	WHITE	SE N2	Field Lab	DESP FL2.2
5	LI HEP 2	ORANGE	LH N2	Field Lab	DESP FL2.2
6	FLUORIDE	YELLOW	F N1	Field Lab	DESP FL2.2

RESPONDENTS AGED 18 mths – 6 yrs

Priority	Blood Tube	Colour	Label Reference	Laboratory	Despatch note
1	EDTA 1	RED	E N1	Addenbrookes	DESP ADDX
2	LI HEP 1	ORANGE	LH N1	Field Lab	DESP FL2.3
3	SERUM 1	BROWN	SE N1	Addenbrookes	DESP ADDX
4	SERUM 2	WHITE	SE N2	Field Lab	DESP FL2.3

CONSENT FORM FOR NDNS

CF (A1)

ADULT AGED 16+

Respondent's name_____(BLOCK LETTERS)

- I have received the information leaflets (Interviewer and Nurse versions) which explain the nature and purpose of the study. I have read and understood these leaflets.
- I am satisfied with any enquiries I have made regarding the study.
- I have been informed that the results will be kept confidential and presented in a way that protects my identity.
- I understand that I may withdraw my consent to any or all of the survey elements at any time without needing to give a reason.

I hereby consent to the following aspects of the study:

BLOOD PRESSURE (TO GP) CONSENT:

Please initial box if consent given

[ ] The survey team sending my blood pressure measurement to my GP.

BMI (TO GP) CONSENT:

Please initial box if consent given

[ ] The survey team sending my body mass index (BMI) measurements to my GP.

24 HOUR URINE CONSENTS:

Please initial box if consent given

[ ] Taking PABA tablets to support the 24-hour urine collection.

[ ] Laboratory analysis of my 24-hour urine collection, to help assess my diet.

[ ] Storage of any remaining urine for tests in the future relating to nutrition and health, provided that the tests are approved by an NHS ethics committee. I understand that I can withdraw my consent to store my urine at any time, without giving any reason, by asking the investigators in writing for my urine to be removed from storage and destroyed. I understand that my data is being used in anonymised form only.

Signature: ....Date ....

CONSENT FORM FOR NDNS

CF (A2)

ADULT AGED 16+

Respondent's name_____(BLOCK LETTERS)

- I have received the information leaflets (Interviewer and Nurse versions) which explain the nature and purpose of the study. I have read and understood these leaflets.

- I am satisfied with any enquiries I have made regarding the study.

- I have been informed that the results will be kept confidential and presented in a way that protects my identity.

- I understand that I may withdraw my consent to any or all of the survey elements at any time without needing to give a reason.

I hereby consent to the following aspects of the study:

BLOOD SAMPLING CONSENTS:

Please initial box if consent given

☐	Having a blood sample for tests related to nutrition and health. This blood sample will not be used for HIV or genetic testing.
☐	<u>I would like</u> / <u>would not like</u> *(delete as appropriate)* to receive a written report of my clinically relevant blood results*.
☐	The NDNS team sending my potentially clinically relevant blood results to my GP*.
☐	Storage of any remaining blood for tests in the future relating to nutrition and health, provided that the tests are approved by an NHS ethics committee. I understand that I can withdraw my consent to store my blood at any time, without giving any reason, by asking the investigators in writing for my blood to be removed from storage and destroyed. I understand that my data is being used in anonymised form only.

*Please note that if you do not want to receive a report of your blood results **and** do not want results to be passed on to your GP we need you to sign a disclaimer (page 6).

Signature: ………………………………………………Date …………………….…

CONSENT FORM FOR NDNS

CHILDREN AGED 4 TO 15 YEARS

Parent/Guardian Section

I agree for my child to participate in the above named survey and in doing so acknowledge that:

- I have received the information leaflets (Interviewer and Nurse versions) which explain the nature and purpose of the study. I have read and understood these leaflets.

- I am satisfied with any enquiries I have made regarding the study.

- I have been informed that the results will be kept confidential and presented in a way that protects my child's identity.

- I understand that I may withdraw my consent to any or all of the survey elements at any time without needing to give a reason.

I hereby agree for my child to participate in the following aspects of the survey:

BLOOD PRESSURE (TO GP) CONSENT:

Please initial box if consent given

[ ] The survey team sending his/her blood pressure measurement to his/her GP.

24 HOUR URINE CONSENTS:

Please initial box if consent given

[ ] Taking PABA tablets to support the 24-hour urine collection.

[ ] Laboratory analysis of his/her 24-hour urine collection, to help assess his/her diet.

[ ] Storage of any remaining urine for tests in the future relating to nutrition and health, provided that the tests are approved by an NHS ethics committee. I understand that I can withdraw my consent to store my child's urine at any time, without giving any reason, by asking the investigators in writing for his/her urine to be removed from storage and destroyed. I understand that my data is being used in anonymised form only.

Respondent's (Child's) Name:……………………………………………………………………………..

Parent/Guardian Name: ……………………………………………………………………………….

Parent/Guardian signature: ………………………………………………Date …………………….

Child assent

I agree to take part in the NDNS survey. I understand the measurements that will be made.

Respondent (Child) signature: ………………………………………………Date…………………….

CONSENT FORM FOR NDNS

CHILDREN AGED 4 TO 15 YEARS

Parent/Guardian Section

I agree for my child to participate in the above named survey and in doing so acknowledge that:

- I have received the information leaflets (Interviewer and Nurse versions) which explain the nature and purpose of the study. I have read and understood these leaflets.

- I am satisfied with any enquiries I have made regarding the study.

- I have been informed that the results will be kept confidential and presented in a way that protects my child's identity.

- I understand that I may withdraw my consent to any or all of the survey elements at any time without needing to give a reason.

- I have been given written information about the Ametop gel and the nurse has explained the purpose and use of Ametop gel to me.

I hereby agree for my child to participate in the following aspects of the survey:

BLOOD SAMPLING CONSENTS:

**Please initial box if consent given**

☐	Blood sample for tests related to nutrition and health. This blood sample will not be used for HIV or genetic testing. Please tick the appropriate box: ☐ with Ametop gel ☐ without Ametop gel
☐	I would like / would not like (delete as appropriate) to receive a written report of my child's clinically relevant blood results*.
☐	The NDNS team sending potentially clinically relevant blood results to his/her GP*.
☐	Storage of any remaining blood for tests in the future relating to nutrition and health, provided that the tests are approved by an NHS ethics committee. I understand that I can withdraw my consent to store my child's blood at any time, without giving any reason, by asking the investigators in writing for his/her blood to be removed from storage and destroyed. I understand that my data is being used in anonymised form only.

*Please note that if you do not want to receive a report of your child's blood results **and** do not want results to be passed on to his/her GP we need you to sign a disclaimer (page 6).

Respondent's (Child's) Name:………………………………………………………………………..

Parent/Guardian Name: ……………………………………………………………………………….

Parent/Guardian signature: ………………………………………………………Date …………………………

Child assent

I agree to take part in the NDNS survey. I understand the measurements that will be made.

Respondent (Child) signature: ………………………………………………………Date……………………

CONSENT FORM FOR NDNS

CHILDREN AGED 1.5 TO 3 YEARS

Parent/Guardian Section

I agree for my child to participate in the above named survey and in doing so acknowledge that:

- I have received the information leaflets (Interviewer and Nurse versions) which explain the nature and purpose of the study. I have read and understood these leaflets.

- I am satisfied with any enquiries I have made regarding the study.

- I have been informed that the results will be kept confidential and presented in a way that protects my child's identity.

- I understand that I may withdraw my consent to any or all of the study elements at any time without needing to give a reason.

- I have been given written information about the Ametop gel and the nurse has explained the purpose and use of Ametop gel to me.

I hereby agree for my child to participate in the following aspects of the study:

BLOOD SAMPLING CONSENTS:

Please initial box if consent given

[ ] Blood sample for tests related to nutrition and health. This blood sample will not be used for HIV or genetic testing. Please tick the appropriate box:

   [ ] with Ametop gel   [ ] without Ametop gel

[ ] I would like / would not like *(delete as appropriate)* to receive a written report of my child's clinically relevant blood results*.

[ ] The NDNS team sending potentially clinically relevant blood results to his/her GP*.

[ ] Storage of any remaining blood for tests in the future relating to nutrition and health, provided that the tests are approved by an NHS ethics committee. I understand that I can withdraw my consent to store my child's blood at any time, without giving any reason, by asking the investigators in writing for his/her blood to be removed from storage and destroyed. I understand that my data is being used in anonymised form only.

*Please note that if you do not want to receive a report of his/her blood results **and** do not want results to be passed on to his/her GP we need you to sign a disclaimer (page 6).

Respondent's (Child's) Name:...

Parent/Guardian Name: ....

Parent/Guardian signature: ....Date ....

NDNS DISCLAIMER

Date:.........................

Name:.. (Block letters)

Respondent's name: .... (Block letters)
(if different from above)

This is to clarify that against the advice of the NDNS survey team I:

Please initial boxes

☐   Do not want to receive <u>my</u> / <u>my child's</u> *(delete as appropriate)* clinically relevant examination results

☐   Do not want <u>my</u> / <u>my child's</u> *(delete as appropriate)* clinically relevant examination results being sent to <u>my</u> / <u>his/her</u> *(delete as appropriate)* GP

I do understand that if there are findings outside the normal range this will not be brought to the attention of any health care provider.

By doing so, I assume all responsibility for my act.

Signed:...

Nurse:...

Nurses - fill in sections in bold <u>only</u>

Volunteer Details

Surname	HNR (use top 9 digit number of label)
Firstname	P952
DOB	/ / dd/mm/yyyy
Sex	**Male** 1
	Female 2 circle as appropriate

Affix serial number label

AddxB1(11)
or
AddxB2 (12)
or
AddxB3 (13)

Study Details

Consultant	JMHNR
Location	NDNS
Title	NDNS
Contact	Katie Dearnley
	01223 426356
Contact OOH	Dr Jennifer Mindell
	020 7679 1269

Sample Details

Date	/ / dd/mm/yyyy	**Volunteer Fasted**	**Yes 1**	
Time	: 24hr clock		**No 2**	circle as appropriate

Sample Tube			Tests	Lab order	Lab barcode	Lab processing
Serum SE1 brown	**Full**	circle as appropriate	Creatinine CRP Lipid Profile TSH Free T4 Free T3	CP952	BIOCHEM BARCODE EDTA sample must be labelled with both biochem & haem barcodes	Automation rack
	Partial					
EDTA EN1 red	**Full**	circle as appropriate	HbA1c Red Cell Folate			Pass to Endo Staff for division of EDTA - instructions below
	Partial		FBC	HA952	HAEM BARCODE	

EDTA separation

Depending on sample volume split the whole blood in the following priority

FBC

Minimum volume required is 1ml – there will be three options:
- Volume less than 1ml (e.g. partial sample) proceed to folate aliquoting and add Meditech comment HAZINS against the haem barcode
- Volume very close to 1ml send primary tube to Haem with the pink duplicate request form, add Meditech comment CCOM and free text against the biochem barcode
- Volume more than ~1.7ml proceed to aliquoting whole blood for folate then primary tube to Haem with the pink duplicate request form

Folate

Take 2x 2ml tubes of ascorbic acid from the bottom half of the -80°C Protect freezer and defrost. Each contains 1ml ascorbic acid – check it has not expired
Print patient biochem barcodes (screen 66)
Label 2x defrosted 2ml ascorbic acid tubes with patient biochem barcodes
Invert the primary EDTA tube a few times to re-suspend the contents
Transfer exactly 100µl from primary EDTA tube into each tube containing 1ml ascorbic acid and invert to mix
Store in the -80°C Protect freezer
If there is sufficient volume proceed to aliquoting whole blood for A1c
If there is insufficient volume left for A1c add a Meditech comment CCOM and free text against the biochem barcode

HbA1c

Label 1x 2ml secondary tube with patient biochem barcode and write A1c
Invert the primary EDTA tube a few times to re-suspend the contents
Transfer 0.5ml from primary EDTA tube into secondary tube
Place secondary tube in A1c skip in office

BLOOD SAMPLE DESPATCH NOTE – FIELD LAB 1 (16+)   DESP FL 2.1

SECTION 1: NURSE complete _all_ sections CLEARLY & LEGIBLY. Enclose with samples to Field Lab

1. Respondent Details

   ```
   Please affix serial
   number label here

   label FL2 (14)
   ```

2. Record respondents sex:

   Male: | 1 |

   Female: | 2 |

3. Was the respondent:

   Fasted | 1 |

   Non-fasted | 2 |

4. Date sample taken: Day [ ][ ]   Month [ ][ ]   Year [ ][ ][ ][ ]

5. Time sample taken: 24 hr clock [ ][ ] : [ ][ ]

6. Time sample delivered to lab: 24 hr clock [ ][ ] : [ ][ ]

7. Nurse Number   [ ][ ][ ][ ][ ][ ]

SECTION 2:   TO BE COMPLETED BY THE FIELD LABORATORY

A. Date sample arrived: Day [ ][ ]   Month [ ][ ]   Year [ ][ ][ ][ ]

B. Time of arrival   24 hr clock [ ][ ] : [ ][ ]

C. Complete table below:

Samples expected:	Sample received?		Volume receiv'd?	Are tubes damaged?	
	Yes	No	mls	Yes	No
EDTA (Red Top) 2.6ml (E N2)					
LiHep 1 (Orange Top) 7.5ml (LH N1)					
LiHep 2 (Orange Top) 7.5ml (LH N2)					
LiHep 3 (Orange Top) 4.5ml (LH N3)					
Plain Serum (White top) 4.5ml (SE N2)					
Fluoride (Yellow top) 1.2ml (F N1)					

Lab technician/analyst:

Please transfer 1300µl whole blood from the well mixed LH N3 tube to the blue capped storage tube (label: LH WB) before starting centrifugation. Place aliquot on ice if not transferred to freezer immediately.

D. Centrifuge tubes as described in the protocol and then complete the following table:

Sample	Time tube centrifuged (24hr clock)	Is the sample abnormal?		If abnormal, code reason _(enter code from list)_
		Yes	No	
E N2	:			
LH N1	:			
LH N2	:			
LH N3	:			
SE N2	:			
F N1	:			

Code frame for abnormal samples:

1 = Haemolysed
2 = Turbid
3 = Lipemic
4 = Frozen
5 = Clot Present (EDTA/LiHep only)
6 = Entirely clotted (EDTA/LiHep only)
7 = Not Clotted (plain serum only)
8 = Other (please describe overleaf)

If other abnormality, please describe here:

E. Please complete table:

Sample	Required Vol (μl)	Actual Vol(μl)	Time of aliquoting	Time of entry into freezer
LH 1	800			
LH 2	800			
LH VITC	300			
LH 3	800			
LH 4	200			
LH 5	400			
LH 6	400			
LH 7	500			
LH 8*	1500			
LH 9*	600 - 1200			
E 1	1000			
SE 1	600			
SE 2*	600			
SE 3*	600			
F 1	500			
LHWB (from LH N3)	1300			
LHN1 washed RBC's	N/A	N/A	N/A	
LHN2 washed RBC's	N/A	N/A	N/A	
LHN3 washed RBC's	N/A	N/A	N/A	

*Please use the remaining plasma to fill LH8 and LH9. Use the remaining serum to fill SE2 and SE3. It is anticipated that there **will not always** be sufficient plasma/serum to fill to the desirable volume. If plasma from either of the LiHep tubes is haemolysed use the clear plasma to fill priority tubes, and the haemolysed plasma to fill the remaining tubes. But always use LiHep plasma from LH N1 or LH N2 (trace metal monovettes) to fill LH5 and LH6. If you have to use LH N3 plasma for LH5 and LH6 then please make a note in the table above.

F. Record temperature samples stored at: _____ °C

G. Sign form - Analyst/Technician sign form:_____ (signature)

_____ (Print name)

BLOOD SAMPLE DESPATCH NOTE – FIELD LAB 1 (aged 7-15)   DESP FL2.2

SECTION 1: NURSE complete <u>all</u> sections CLEARLY & LEGIBLY. Enclose with samples to Field Lab

1.   Respondent Details

Please affix serial
number label here

Label FL2(14)

2.   Record respondents sex:

Male:	1
Female:	2

3.   Was the respondent:

Fasted	1
Non-fasted	2

4.   Date sample taken:

Day		Month		Year			

5.   Time sample taken: 24 hr clock
[ ][ ] : [ ][ ]

6.   Time sample delivered to lab: 24 hr clock
[ ][ ] : [ ][ ]

7.   Nurse Number
[ ][ ][ ][ ][ ][ ]

SECTION 2:   TO BE COMPLETED BY THE FIELD LABORATORY

A.   Date sample arrived:

Day		Month		Year			

B.   Time of arrival   24 hr clock
[ ][ ] : [ ][ ]

C.   Complete table below:

Samples expected:	Sample received?		Volume receiv'd?	Are tubes damaged?	
	Yes	**No**	**mls**	**Yes**	**No**
LiHep 1 (Orange Top) 7.5ml (LH N1)					
LiHep 2 (Orange Top) 2.7ml (LH N2)					
Plain Serum (White top) 4.5ml (SE N2)					
Fluoride (Yellow top) 1.2ml (F N1)					

D.   Centrifuge tubes as described in the protocol and then complete the following table:

Sample	Time tube centrifuged (24hr clock)	Is the sample abnormal?		If abnormal, code reason *(enter code from list)*
		Yes	**No**	
LH N1	:			
LH N2	:			
SE N2	:			
F N1	:			

Code frame for abnormal samples:

1 = Haemolysed
2 = Turbid
3 = Lipemic
4 = Frozen
5 = Clot Present (EDTA/LiHep only)
6 = Entirely clotted (EDTA/LiHep only)
7 = Not Clotted (plain serum only)
8 = Other (please describe overleaf)

If other abnormality, please describe here:

E. Please complete table:

Sample	Required Vol (μl)	Actual Vol(μl)	Time of aliquoting	Time of entry into freezer
LH 1	600			
LH 2	800			
LH VITC	300			
LH 3	800			
LH 4	300			
LH 5	200			
LH 6	500			
LH 7	300			
SE 1	600			
SE 2	600			
SE 3	600			
F 1	500			
LHN1 washed RBCs	N/A	N/A	N/A	
LH N2 washed RBCs	N/A	N/A	N/A	

If plasma from either of the LiHep tubes is haemolysed use the clear plasma to fill priority tubes, and the haemolysed plasma to fill the remaining tubes. But always use LiHep plasma from LH N1 (trace metal monovette) to fill LH4. If you have to use LH N2 plasma for LH4 then please make a note in the table above.

F. Record temperature samples stored at: _____°C

G. Sign form - Analyst/Technician sign form:_____ (signature)

_____ (Print name)

This record must **be faxed to HNR** on the day of sample processing:
Fax No.: **01223 437546**

The original must be returned to HNR with the samples and spare labels via courier at the pre-arranged date.

BLOOD SAMPLE DESPATCH NOTE – FIELD LAB 1 (18mths – 6yrs)   DESP FL2.3

SECTION 1: NURSE complete <u>all</u> sections CLEARLY & LEGIBLY. Enclose with samples to Field Lab

1. Respondent Details

> Please affix serial number label here
>
> **Label FL2**(14)

2. Record respondents sex:

Male: | 1
Female: | 2

3. Was the respondent:

Fasted | 1
Non-fasted | 2

4. Date sample taken: Day   Month   Year

5. Time sample taken: 24 hr clock

6. Time sample delivered to lab: 24 hr clock

7. Nurse Number

SECTION 2: TO BE COMPLETED BY THE FIELD LABORATORY

A. Date sample arrived: Day   Month   Year

B. Time of arrival   24 hr clock

C. Complete table below:

Samples expected:	Sample received?		Volume receiv'd?	Are tubes damaged?	
	Yes	**No**	**mls**	**Yes**	**No**
LiHep (Orange Top) 4.5ml (LH N1)					
Plain Serum (White top) 2.7ml (SE N2)					

D. Centrifuge tubes as described in the protocol and then complete the following table:

Sample	Time tube centrifuged (24hr clock)	Is the sample abnormal?		If abnormal, code reason *(enter code from list)*
		Yes	**No**	
LH N1	:			
SE N2	:			

Code frame for abnormal samples:

1 = Haemolysed
2 = Turbid
3 = Lipemic
4 = Frozen
5 = Clot Present (EDTA/LiHep only)
6 = Entirely clotted (EDTA/LiHep only)
7 = Not Clotted (plain serum only)
8 = Other (please describe overleaf)

If other abnormality, please describe here:

E. Please complete table:

Sample	Required Vol (µl)	Actual Vol (µl)	Time of aliquoting	Time of entry into freezer
LH 1	400			
LH 2	600			
LH VITC	300			
LH 3	500			
SE 1	600			
SE 2	400			
LHN1 washed RBCs	N/A	N/A	N/A	

F. Record temperature samples stored at: _____ °C

G. Sign form - Analyst/Technician sign form:_____ (signature)

_____ (Print name)

This record must **be faxed to HNR** on the day of sample processing:
Fax No.: **01223 437546**

The original must be returned to HNR with the samples and spare labels via courier at the pre-arranged date.

To be completed by the nurse

Nurse Name [   ]

Nurse Number [ ][ ][ ][ ][ ][ ]

1. **Respondent details**

[
Please affix serial
number label here

Label UDESP(36)
]

Please complete one record for each respondent.

Q1 Did the respondent consent to taking PABA tablets?

Yes [ ]
No [ ]

Q2 Did the respondent consent to the storage of any remaining urine?

Yes [ ]
No [ ]

Q3 Was there any urine inside the 2L bottle?

Yes [ ] Weigh BOTH the 2L and 5L bottles separately BEFORE mixing together (if possible) to sub sample the urine. Record 5 litre weights at **Q4** and 2 litre weights at **Q5**.

No [ ] Weigh the 5L bottle only. Record weights below (**Q4**).

Q4 **Type of container:** [ ] **5.0L** jerry can

- Weigh the urine a **first time**, on the digital scales provided, and record the weight in **kilograms** of the 5L bottle containing the urine:

[__ __ . __] **kg**

- Weigh the urine a **second time** and record the weight in **kilograms** of the 5L bottle containing the urine:

[__ __ . __] **kg**

- If the first and second weights differ by more than 0.02kg weigh the urine a **third time** and record the weight in **kilograms** of the 5L bottle containing the urine:

[|]   **kg**

If no urine in 2L bottle: mix the urine and take **4 sub-samples** and discard the remaining urine nd equipment as per instructions provided. **If any urine in 2L bottle: go to Q5.**

Q5. **Type of container:** [   ] **2.0L** jerry can

- Weigh the urine a **first time**, on the digital scales provided, and record the weight in **kilograms** of the 2L bottle containing the urine:

[|]   **kg**

- Weigh the urine a **second time** and record the weight in **kilograms** of the 2L bottle containing the urine:

[|]   **kg**

- If the first and second weights differ by more than 0.02kg weigh the urine a **third time** and record the weight in **kilograms** of the 2L bottle containing the urine:

[|]   **kg**

Q6. Can all urine in the 2L bottle be transferred into the 5L bottle?

Yes [   ]   Go to Q7
No   [   ]   Go to Q8

Q7. Weigh first, then transfer urine from 2L bottle to 5L bottle. Mix urine before sub-sampling from 5L bottle **only**: mix the urine and take **4 sub-samples** and discard the remaining urine and equipment as per instructions provided.

Q8. If urine collected in 2L bottle will not fit in 5L bottle, do not transfer. Note the weight of the 2L bottle above but **only** sub-sample from 5L bottle: mix the urine and take **4 sub-samples** and discard the remaining urine and equipment as per instructions provided.

Please use the packaging provided to send the following items to HNR:
- **one copy of the respondent 24-hour urine collection sheet**
- **the completed urine volume and dispatch sheet**
- **and the urine sub-samples**

Please post the packet of samples as soon as possible in a post-box;
check for same day collection.

DESPATCH NOTE FOR ALL SAMPLES

DESP OFFICE

(OFFICE COPY)

1. Respondent Details

```
┌─────────────────────────────┐
│                             │
│  Please affix serial number │
│        label here           │
│                             │
│    Label OFFDESP (2)        │
│                             │
│                             │
└─────────────────────────────┘
```

Circle one code only

Samples obtained: *(tick all that apply)*

2. Age group:

16+ **1** — EDTA 1 ☐ EDTA 2 ☐ Serum 1 ☐ Serum 2 ☐ Li Hep1 ☐
Li Hep2 ☐ Li Hep3 ☐ Fluoride ☐ 24 hr Urine ☐

7-15 **2** — EDTA 1 ☐ Serum1 ☐ Serum 2 ☐ Li Hep 1 ☐ Li Hep2 ☐
Fluoride ☐ 24 hr Urine ☐

4-6 **3** — EDTA 1 ☐ Serum1 ☐ Serum 2 ☐ Li Hep 1 ☐ 24 hr Urine ☐

18 mths – 3 yrs **4** — EDTA 1 ☐ Serum1 ☐ Serum 2 ☐ Li Hep 1 ☐

3. Date blood sample taken:
Day ☐☐ Month ☐☐ Year ☐☐☐☐

4. Time Blood sample taken:
24 hr clock ☐☐ : ☐☐

5. Date blood despatched to Addenbrookes:
Day ☐☐ Month ☐☐ Year ☐☐☐☐

6. Date Urine sub-sampled:
Day ☐☐ Month ☐☐ Year ☐☐☐☐

7. Did you experience any problems in taking the Venepuncture? If yes, please record these below and state what action you took. (PROMPTED FROM CAPI)